Care of the Older Adult

Care of the Older Adult

JOAN BIRCHENALL R.N., M. Ed.

Director of Health Occupations Education
New Jersey Department of Education
Trenton, New Jersey

MARY EILEEN STREIGHT R.N., B.S.N.

Lecturer
Office of Vocational Education
Department of Industrial Education and Technology
Trenton, New Jersey

J. B. LIPPINCOTT COMPANY
Philadelphia   Toronto

Distributed in Great Britain
Blackwell Scientific Publications, Oxford, London, and Edinburgh

ISBN 0-397-54129-5
Library of Congress Catalog Card Number 73-6834
Printed in the United States of America
3 5 7 9 8 6 4 2

Library of Congress Cataloging in Publication Data

Birchenall, Joan.
    Care of the Older Adult.
    Includes bibliographies.

    1. Geriatric nursing.   I. Streight, Mary Eileen, joint author.   II Title.   (DNLM:

    1. Geriatric nursing.   WY152 B617c   1973)

RC954.B57   610.73'65   73-6834

ISBN 0-397-54129-5

*To our families
for their patience, sacrifice, understanding
and support*

Preface

Increased numbers of nursing homes, extended care facilities, and new legislation for older Americans have brought the senior citizen and his needs into sharper focus.

Allied health personnel are being utilized in health care facilities to provide the bulk of geriatric care. *Care of the Older Adult* has been written to fill a growing need for a text that is suitable for use by practical nurses and allied health personnel. Competent geriatric care is built on an understanding of the normal process of aging and of the developmental tasks of the late adult years.

The text includes suggestions for using this understanding as a basis for nursing care of the aged. Emphasis is placed on the role the nurse can play in the preventive aspects of geriatric care and in the process of restorative nursing. No attempt has been made to include fundamentals of nursing, since it is assumed that the reader has necessary skills and an understanding of these fundamentals. Modification of nursing techniques to meet the needs of the patient requiring long-term care has been integrated into the text.

It is further assumed that the reader has a knowledge of normal body structure and functions, community health, nutrition, working relationships, and other areas basic to the practical nursing and allied health personnel curricula. The questions and problems at the end of each chapter provide an opportunity for the student to apply knowledge acquired in previous courses, such as medical-surgical nursing and psychiatric nursing, to the care of the aged.

The beginning of the book provides general background information on the aging population in the United States. Attitudes of various ethnic groups toward the aged and those arising from our youth-oriented culture are discussed. The needs of the aging, including social, emotional, economic, and spiritual needs, have been incorporated, and the latest available information on federal and state legislation concerning older Americans is given.

Next the book discusses the normal aging process and how to cope with it. Approaches to the problems that are caused by the aging process are suggested.

The text then discusses the nursing of patients requiring long-term care. The disease conditions included were selected because of the high incidence found in the aged population.

Finally, the book looks to the reader's future. The importance of planning for one's later years is stressed, and practical guidelines for a healthy, well-adjusted retirement are incorporated. Consideration is given to the possible influence of technological advances on geriatric care in the future.

Throughout this text the authors have endeavored to demonstrate their philosophy that the aging process need not be feared. It is their belief that understanding the problems of late adulthood and planning for this phase of one's life are essential to the enjoyment of the "leisure years." For these reasons the authors have utilized positive approaches to the aging process and geriatric nursing care.

Acknowledgments

The authors are most grateful to the many people who gave invaluable assistance to them in the preparation of the manuscript. Special thanks is given to Elizabeth V. Moore, R.N., Consultant, Health Careers, New Jersey Department of Education, and Susan B. Glocke, R.P.T., Consultant, Comprehensive Health Planning, New Jersey Department of Health, for their suggestions concerning the content, and to Margaret B. Birchenall who provided the research assistance needed to write the manuscript.

The following individuals and agencies provided illustrations and photographs: John Leahy, photographer; Donald Vannozzi, artist; Morris Hall Health and Rehabilitation Center, Lawrenceville, New Jersey; Visiting Nurse Association of Trenton, New Jersey; and Green Thumb, Inc., Trenton, New Jersey.

Mary Ann Ryan, Helen Hritz, and Anne J. Ryan provided their clerical skills in the preparation of the manuscript. Our sincere thanks to Michaelene Paulick for typing and proofreading the major portion of the material.

Finally, the authors wish to express their gratitude to David T. Miller, J. B. Lippincott Company, for his suggestions, support, and encouragement.

Contents

1

The Aging Population

At the turn of the century one out of twenty-five Americans was age sixty-five or over. Now this ratio has increased to one out of ten. Each year approximately 1.4 million persons reach their sixty-fifth birthday. It is estimated that by the year 2000 this population will reach the 32 million mark (Figure 1-1).

This growth reflects the increase in average life expectancy rates. In 1900 the average life expectancy was forty-three years. Today the average life expectancy for a man celebrating his sixty-fifth birthday is seventy-eight years of age, and women have a three-year edge over men. Generally, white people have a higher life expectancy than the nonwhite population. The real significance of the growth of the population group over sixty-five, however, is the number of people living beyond the average life expectancy.

UNDER AGE 45	45-64 YEARS	65 AND OVER
69%	21%	10%

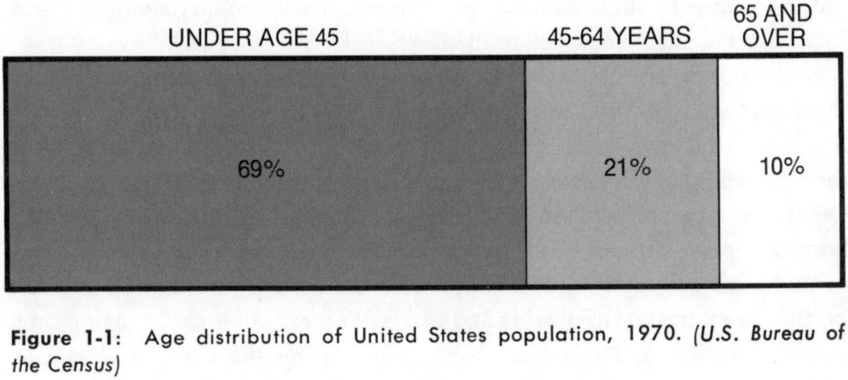

Figure 1-1: Age distribution of United States population, 1970. *(U.S. Bureau of the Census)*

1

Of the 20 million persons who are sixty-five or over, about 10 million are under seventy-three. However, 1.3 million persons are eighty-five or older. If current trends continue, the population of those who are eighty-five or older may well double. This has real implications for the kind and quality of health care that should be available to this age group, in which physical disability and disease conditions become increasingly more prevalent. Experts in the field are now classifying the old into two categories—the "younger" old and the "older" old. The needs of the two groups are distinct, and in the planning of health care the unique needs of each group must be considered.

To each person the term "old" has a different meaning. To the child "old" may mean a chronological age of twenty. To the teen-ager anyone over thirty is "over the hill." To the person aged seventy-five "old" means anyone older than himself! We tend to associate "oldness" with infirmity and decrepitude but this is not necessarily the case. Our society has many false notions about aging. The advanced years are viewed as stealers of all those qualities that we strive so to attain, including the zest for life, robust health, and total involvement in the world around us—the ability to be an active contributor to the great American way of life. When the magic age of sixty-five arrives, however, we expect all sorts of unpleasant phenomena suddenly to occur—age descends; the curtain falls; the golden age proves to be a myth. The active contributor now becomes the passive receiver of whatever an ungrateful society leaves for him, a second-class citizen. How wrong these statements are, but unfortunately such attitudes color our relationships with the elderly and build barriers to mutual respect and understanding.

Aging is a process or series of processes that begins at conception. Of course, the rate at which body tissues, organs, and systems age varies, with more rapid and noticeable changes taking place during the later years. Still the rate of change differs with each individual. The inevitable aging process is highly individualized and encompasses the psychological and social aspects of aging as well as the biological.

We still do not know the precise causes of aging, but gerontologists, or those who study the multiple aspects of aging, are trying to find the answer. Some gerontologists believe that the process most likely to cause aging is the toughening of connective tissue, or collagen, and other fibrous proteins. Others feel that the answer to the secret of aging lies in the role that the hormones play. Although long-range research on aging requires generations of study, research findings will continue to yield much information that can be applied to the field of nursing and particularly gerontological nursing care.

One's personality is not changed merely by his chronological age.

Unless his personality has been altered by pathological changes in the body, he will be "the same" as he always was. The trite labels applied to older people are false and sometimes degrading. The phrase "back to childhood" connotes the idea that elderly persons must be treated as children. The comments "rigid" and "unable to adapt" suggest that they are beyond changing. The inevitable physical changes accompanying the aging process, coupled with the many misconceptions concerning behavioral patterns, lead to the social isolation of the older person. Our society, preoccupied with maintaining youth, regards retirement as the end of a productive life and the aged as a burden to be tolerated or to be cared for in institutions.

Our views of aging and older persons are dependent on our own personal experiences with relatives, friends, and acquaintances. Our cultural and ethnic backgrounds play a role in the formation of our ideas and opinions. Today, the focus is on youth. The advertising industry directs its campaigns at the young or those who wish to identify with youth. We are also a work-oriented society, in which work is considered honorable and acceptable, and leisure, in order to be acceptable, must be earned. Leisure is viewed as a precious time between intervals of productivity—a time for the worker to renew mind and body so that he can return to work refreshed. The retiree's leisure time, however, is classified as nonproductive and therefore lacking in social value. Perhaps, these views are the result of a culture that has been based on building a nation, the backbone of which is a working class of people who, up until recent years, died before ever reaching old age. Never before have there been so many aged persons, so many retirees.

In many instances older adults do not live with other family members or even near to them (Figure 1-2). The family, rather than being a closely knit unit, is scattered. Children, therefore, do not have an opportunity to grow up with older relatives and to develop positive attitudes toward them. In some societies the elderly are regarded with great respect and honor. For example, in traditional China the aged were respected for the wisdom they had accrued during a long lifetime. Responsibility for elderly parents automatically became the duty of the eldest son. Other ethnic groups are also known for their careful attention to the needs—physical, social, and spiritual—of their older members. The customs of these groups, however, are often missing in second-, third-, and fourth-generation Americans. Somehow, in our haste to build a better world, we have forgotten the mark of a caring society—preservation of the dignity of its older citizens.

It is impossible to generalize about the life-style of the elderly—their living accommodations, income, nutrition, and so on. However, the following information may present a picture of some of the problems the elderly face in adapting to today's society.

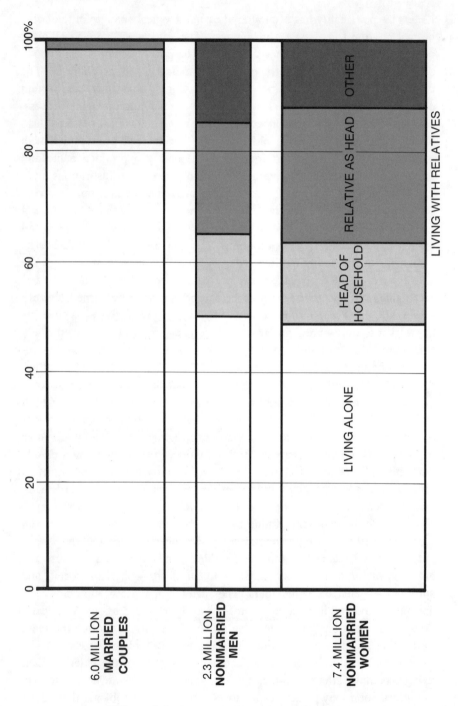

Figure 1-2: Living arrangements of the aged.

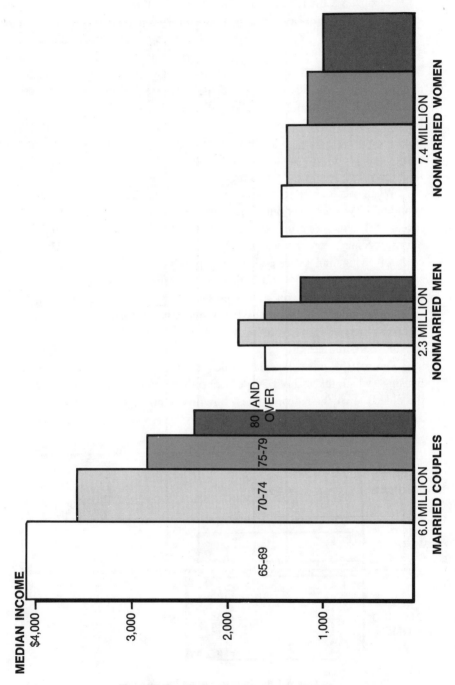

Figure 1-3: Median income by age.

Because of their contacts with hospitalized patients, nurses tend to categorize the elderly as a group whose main characteristic is illness and resulting disability. This false impression can color the nurse's attitude and approach to the elderly person. Although recent studies have shown that 86 percent of the 20 million older Americans have some impairment, chronic illness, or disease, only 5 percent are hospitalized or institutionalized. It has also been estimated that almost half of those institutionalized are misplaced or could be cared for in a more appropriate non-institutionalized setting if such were available. This indicates that the elderly, as a group, are able to adapt to physical impairments more readily than the young would like to admit.

When we look at the income levels of the aged, we find that this adaptability carries over into the economic sector. Most recent statistics reveal that almost one quarter of the total elderly population (5 million), has an income below the designated poverty level (Figure 1-3). The rising costs of living and decreased buying power of the dollar force a tight squeeze on the pocketbook for those dependent on a fixed retirement income. A widow living on a budget of $32 per week certainly must be highly adaptable in order to survive. Obviously, this limited income affects the older person's ability to provide for the most basic human needs— shelter, food, and health.

One of the most expensive budget items the aged must consider is housing (which takes about 34 percent of his income). About two-thirds of the elderly own their own homes, but this is not always as advantageous as it would seem (Figure 1-4). Not only are taxes rising, but the homeowner

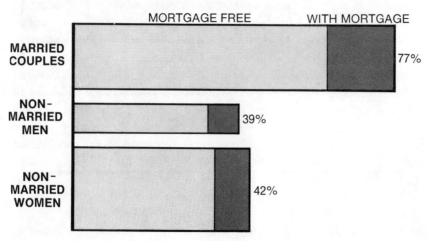

Figure 1-4: Homes owned by the aged.

may have physical limitations that make necessary repairs and adequate maintenance difficult or impossible, forcing him to pay others for essential repairs and upkeep of the home. Many such homeowners live in older neighborhoods of cities, areas that have been hard hit by urban decay. Property that was once valuable has now been devalued to the point where selling the home (if it can be sold) is unwise from a financial viewpoint. Alternatives to home ownership are very limited for those whose income is marginal or at poverty level. The building of low-cost public housing units has not kept pace with the need. It is estimated that 6 million older persons are still in need of decent housing. Escalating rents for sometimes uninhabitable apartments are imposed upon the elderly, who are least able to fight this inhumane treatment. Many reside in single rooms in run-down hotels and boarding houses, which are unhealthy and structurally unsafe, and contribute to the degradation of the aged.

Food represents the next highest budget expenditure. The Bureau of Labor Statistics estimates that approximately 27 percent of the elderly's income goes for food. Spiraling food costs and limited income are only two causes for the high incidence of malnutrition in this age group. In many instances the lack of a nearby grocery store or supermarket, the lack of transportation, and the problem of carrying heavy packages are obstacles that hinder the aged in securing food. The physiological changes and emotional factors that enter into the nutritional problems of the elderly will be discussed in future chapters. Suffice it to say that in this land of plenty the system of delivery of food and goods to the consumer does not provide for the special and individualized needs of our older citizens. If 27 percent of their income is spent on food, then the elderly need to be "consumer wise," so that the dollars they spend yield the greatest benefit. Unfortunately, many pay a higher price than necessary for food and other services because of ignorance regarding their consumer rights.

As has been mentioned, older adults as a group are not as incapacitated by illness as we would think. As age increases, however, the incidence of chronic disease conditions does increase. The inner resources of this age group, however, create the adaptability necessary to weather chronic illness or disability without hospitalization. According to the most recent studies of the National Center for Health Statistics, 15 million noninstitutionalized persons sixty-five or over have at least one chronic disease condition. The activities of 7.5 million members of this group are limited to some extent because of these chronic conditions. Arthritis is by far the biggest culprit. About 80 percent of our older population is affected in some way by this disease. As with the younger population, heart diseases, cancer, and cerebral vascular diseases (predominantly strokes) are the three major causes of death. All three may necessitate long periods of hospitalization, in either an acute hospital, extended care facility, rehabilitation center, or nursing home. When illness strikes the elderly, longer and more frequent hospital stays are the rule rather than the exception. Studies have shown that one person in seven between forty-five and sixty-four is hospitalized per year. For those sixty-five and over the ratio is one person in four. The average length of the hospital stay also rises.

Thus the costs of health care also rise as age increases. The increasing incidence of chronic disease, necessitating doctors' visits, diagnostic tests, therapeutic diets, medications, and longer periods of hospitalization, make health care extremely expensive. One of the real fears of the aged person is that medical expenses will eat away his savings and render him totally dependent. In fiscal year 1971 the average per capita cost of health care, including hospitalization, for those in the sixty-five and over age group was $861. Figure 1-5 shows the comparison of average per capita total health care expenditures for those persons under nineteen, nineteen to sixty-four, and sixty-five and over.

In contrast to the annual expenditure for the elderly, the yearly cost of health care for the young was $140, and for the intermediate age group, $323. A breakdown of the costs for the elderly shows that hospital care, totaling $410, accounted for the greatest bulk of their annual expenditure. The cost for physicians' services was $144, with other services, such as nursing home care, drugs, eyeglasses and other aids, and dentists' services amounting to $307. Although $636 of the total bill was provided by government health insurance and other public sources, $225 had to be paid by the elderly.[1] How easily one's nest egg can vanish as the costs of health care and illness increase. Health care legislation will be discussed in Chapter 3.

The plight of our older population has received considerable publicity in the past decade. Nationally, in 1961 and 1971 our government sponsored two White House conferences on aging. Key issues confronting older Americans were discussed and brought to the public's attention. The 1971 conference was preceded by statewide meetings at which older Americans discussed their needs and problems. When the conference convened, fourteen subject areas were discussed, including the basic human needs (shelter, clothing, food, and health) and ways in which these needs can be satisfied. Hopefully, the ongoing post conferences throughout the 1970s will assure that recommendations are implemented. Our national priorities must be reordered so that the major problems confronting the elderly can

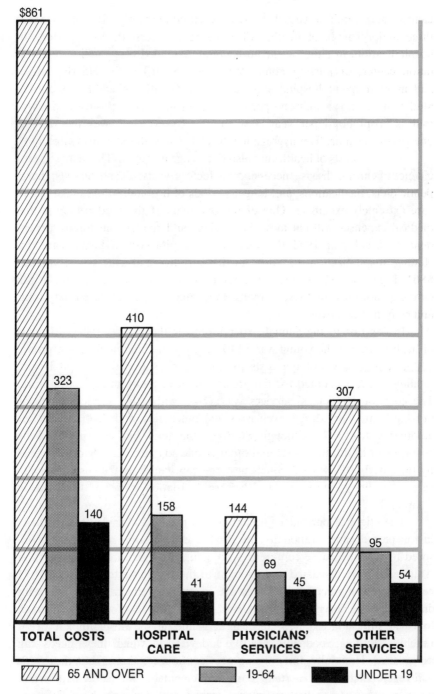

Figure 1-5: 1971 per capita health care costs for three age groups.

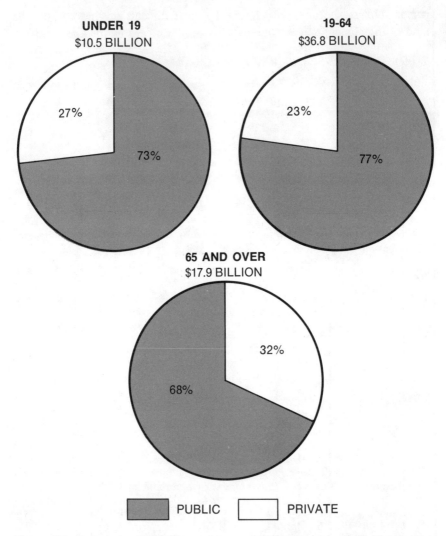

Figure 1-6: Percentage distribution of expenditures for personal health care, by source of funds and by age group, fiscal year 1971.

be overcome, if our older citizens are to be given a chance to live with pride and in dignity.

The provision of health care has continued to be a topic of discussion since the most recent conference. We have been accused of dehumanizing the treatment of the elderly. If we are to correct this and humanize our care, each person must be treated as a unique person, with individual needs, and not simply as another seventy-two-year-old.

The nurse needs to examine her real views on aging and the older person. Unless she does this, it will be most difficult for her to give the kind of individualized care our patients need and are entitled to receive.

STUDY QUESTIONS AND PROBLEMS

1. Do a survey of members in your family or community who are in the following age groups to find out what the word "old" means to them:

10-15	35-50
16-19	50-65
20-25	65 and over
25-35	

2. What are your views on aging and the older adult? Discuss.
3. Discuss the youth-oriented culture in the United States. Bring specific examples to class, such as advertisements, newspaper and magazine articles, and other evidence.
4. Have any steps been taken in your community to implement the recommendations of the White House Conference on Aging?

BIBLIOGRAPHY

A Pre-White House Conference on Aging—Summary of Development and Data. Washington, D.C.: U.S. Government Printing Office, 1971.

Burgess, Ernest W. *Aging in Western Societies.* Chicago: University of Chicago Press, 1960.

de Beauvoir, Simone. *The Coming of Age.* New York: G. P. Putnam's Sons, 1972.

Developments in Aging 1970. Washington, D.C.: U.S. Government Printing Office, 1971.

1971 White House Conference on Aging. Washington, D.C.: U.S. Government Printing Office, 1971.

U.S., Department of Health, Education, and Welfare, *Health in the Later Years of Life.* Washington, D.C.: U.S. Government Printing Office, 1971.

U.S., Department of Health, Education, and Welfare, Social Security Administration, Office of Research and Statistics, *Resources of People 65 or Over.* Washington, D.C.: U.S. Government Printing Office, 1971.

U.S., Department of Health, Education, and Welfare, Social Security Administration, *Social Security Bulletin,* vol. 35, No. 5. DHEW Pub. No. (SSA) 72-11700. Washington, D.C.: U.S. Government Printing Office, May 1972.

U.S., Department of Health, Education, and Welfare, *Working with Older People—A Guide to Practice,* vol. 2, *Biological, Psychological and Sociological Aspects of Aging.* Washington, D.C.: U.S. Government Printing Office, 1970.

U.S., Department of Health, Education, and Welfare, *Working with Older People—A Guide to Practice,* vol. 3, *The Aging Person: Needs and Services.* Washington, D.C.: U.S. Government Printing Office, 1970.

NOTES

1. Barbara Cooper and Nancy Worthington. *Medical Care Spending for Three Age Groups.* U.S. Department of Health, Education, and Welfare, Office of Research and Statistics, Social Security Bulletin. p. 13. Washington, D.C.: U.S. Government Printing Office, May 1972.

2

Developmental Tasks of Older Adults

In every stage of one's life there are certain tasks to be accomplished, things to learn, adjustments to be made, and problems to be solved. Collectively, these are known as developmental tasks. The challenges of developmental tasks for the infant are quite obvious, many of these tasks relating to his adjustment to his own body and his environment. You can easily observe the child who has discovered his hands and inspects these for great lengths of time, not only looking at them but also moving and tasting them.

The developmental tasks accomplished by the aging person are not as readily observable as those accomplished in infancy. However, the tasks facing the older person are no less challenging or crucial. They are a vital part of living.

Evelyn Duvall[1] cites two critical developmental tasks: (a) finding life meaningful after retirement and (b) adjusting to decreasing physical health and strength. Other tasks, which affect one's social, physical, emotional, and economic adjustment, are derived from these basic developmental tasks.

Some older adults choose not to retire from full-time employment. This is especially true of those who are self-employed and work many years beyond retirement age. Their developmental tasks may mean adjusting to diminishing strength and physical health with, perhaps, decreasing active involvement in the business as time goes on. The choice, to retire or not, should be made by the older adult rather than enforced by society's

12

arbitrary rules. The remainder of the chapter deals with the needs of the majority of Americans who retire by will or by request during the later years of life.

RETIREMENT

Many men look forward to retirement as an opportunity to relax and enjoy a life free of set routines, time schedules, and the pressures of work. The period before the last day of work is usually filled with rounds of parties, retirement dinners, and the accepting of tokens of accomplishment from fellow workers and management. These are indeed very busy and exciting times. They may also be spent orienting the new man who will take over the retiree's duties. Cleaning out the desk, tool crib, etc., socializing, and discussing the better days to come are pleasurable. However, while the retiree-to-be is outwardly joking about those better days, he may be inwardly concerned about what his retirement is really going to mean. If he has not adequately prepared himself for this new phase of life, the act of retirement may come as a shock. What will take the place of gainful employment? What will provide a sense of meaning and worthwhile endeavor? The problems of finding life meaningful after retirement, once unique to the male, must also, in these modern times, be faced by the woman who has returned to employment after her children have grown.

After an initial period, when the couple takes long-awaited pleasure trips, they face the problem of extra idle hours each day. How can they remain contributing members of the community?

A Meaningful Life

Some men and women, particularly former executives, continue to act as consultants to their former employers. The company is then provided with the services of key personnel who have an objective viewpoint, and the retired person in turn maintains his sense of usefulness, since he continues to be a contributing member of society. Some retired business leaders belong to associations whose primary objective is to assist novice businessmen in the development of sound business practices.

Many retired persons choose to obtain part-time employment, both as a means of feeling needed and to supplement their retirement incomes. A few of the positions suited to the needs and capabilities of older Americans are school-crossing guards, meter patrolmen, baby-sitters, sales personnel, caterers, and watchmen. The American Association of Retired Persons (AARP) has established an employment service for members who wish to work on a part-time basis. The service, which is called Mature

Temps, was established in 1969 at the request of AARP members and the National Retired Teachers Association. In the first year of operation Mature Temps workers earned $650,000, but the rewards cannot be measured in dollars and cents, for the feeling of usefulness cannot be bought. Information concerning this service can be obtained by contacting Mature Temps, 521 Fifth Avenue, New York, N.Y. 10017.

Some older Americans may prefer volunteer work to part-time employment. Those who have been involved in limited volunteer work throughout their employed lives now have more time to contribute. The person who wishes to become a volunteer may contact the Volunteer Service Bureau in his community. This bureau attempts to match the volunteer's interests, abilities, and skills to the jobs available.

Both the Peace Corps and VISTA (Volunteers in Service to America) accept retired persons with special abilities. The experiences of a lifetime can be shared with fellow Americans or with peoples of new and emerging nations. The work and living conditions are demanding and rigorous, but this will not be a new experience for many retired persons. Information on VISTA and the Peace Corps may be obtained by writing these agencies in Washington, D.C.

One of the most universally available activities is the senior citizen or golden age club. These clubs are operated by churches, community centers, antipoverty agencies, and the recreation departments of local governments. Such clubs are not designed for people who wish to sit in rocking chairs and watch the time pass by. Rather, members participate in community, recreational, and social activities. Some of the community services include making cancer dressings, recording for the blind, tutoring inner-city school children, and acting as grandparents for institutionalized children. Glee clubs, bands and orchestras, dances, art groups, group trips, theater parties, and buffet suppers are examples of social and recreational activities. The benefits of club membership include the opportunity to meet and enjoy old and new friends, group trips at reduced rates, discount cards for local movies, and special fares on public transportation.

Many men and women continue active membership in organizations to which they have already devoted many years, including civic, church, professional, and fraternal associations, political clubs, and hobby and arts-and-crafts groups. Specialized clubs, such as photography, gardening, bridge, and coin- and stamp-collecting clubs, provide opportunities for people to share mutual interests. Some of these clubs offer reduced membership rates for retired persons.

Can an old dog be taught new tricks? Yes, if he wants to learn, and many retired people want to do just that. How many times have you read about a grandmother earning her college diploma or a grandfather graduating from high school? The completion of one's education brings a sense of accomplishment, satisfaction, and pride that cannot be bought or measured and is invaluable at any age.

If the older person wishes to enrich his life and stay up-to-date and informed, he has many resources available. Evening adult schools offer a variety of courses, including preparation for the high-school equivalency examination, gourmet cooking, furniture refinishing, first aid, and golf.

The local Y. usually has a busy schedule of daytime programs, offering courses in arts, crafts, and physical fitness. These subjects are of interest to mature men and women and are offered at a time convenient for them.

The American Association of Retired Persons conducts an Institute of Lifetime Learning, which offers home study courses for AARP members who wish to stay informed.

The Retirement Income

Sometimes retirement income equals the person's employment income, in which case no adjustments may be required. Many times, however, the retirement income may be reduced. Futhermore, it may be a fixed income, and since it does not increase as the cost of living increases, it does not have the same buying power after a few years.

For most retirees the major source of income is Social Security benefits. (Additional information on the Social Security Act may be found in Chapter 3.) If this is the only money coming into the household, the couple will find that its income is quite limited, and many adjustments will have to be made.

Social Security benefits are based on the amount of money the retired person and his employer paid into the fund during his working years. Computation of the husband's retirement income is based on his earnings. If the wife has been gainfully employed for a sufficient length of time, she may collect Social Security benefits from her own earnings. However, she may also collect benefits from her husband's income. She has a choice between collecting from her own or from her husband's Social Security benefits and may choose whichever is greater.

Pension plans provide another source of income. Many businesses offer group retirement funds for their employees. Sometimes the employer contributes money to the fund. Such funds are controlled by a board of trustees or a private insurance company, which is responsible for investing the monies to ensure financial growth through good fiscal policies. Usually, the employee's contribution to the pension plan is deducted directly from his salary, as is his Social Security payment. The longer one belongs to the employee's retirement fund, the more he saves, and the greater his income is upon retirement.

Some retirees have not had the opportunity to participate in employer-sponsored pension plans. There are many reasons for this. Some companies are too small to have an economically sound retirement plan. The person may have been self-employed, or he may have job-hopped, never being employed in one company long enough to participate fully in a retirement plan. Many women who return to gainful employment in their forties and fifties are not eligible for employer-sponsored pension plans because of their age.

Many people caught in these situations have had the foresight to participate in one of the pension plans offered by major insurance companies. The earlier a person joins one of these plans, the smaller the premium and the greater the length of time to save. The individual obtaining the policy must decide how much money to invest in the plan, which he does with the consultation of his insurance agent. Premium payments terminate after a specified time (stipulated in the insurance policy), and the benefits usually begin upon retirement. Some labor unions and professional associations offer participation in such plans at reduced rates for their members.

Investments represent another source of income for retirees. These may be savings accounts, stocks and bonds, or government securities. However, the investment holdings should be large enough for the interest to provide a good income. If the investments themselves must be tapped, they then represent a dwindling income that cannot be relied on as a constant source of money. Many retired persons look upon their investment holdings as a source of emergency money—for medical bills in the event of an overwhelming illness or for major unexpected repairs on their home or car.

All kinds of retirement incomes, then, are the result of a lifetime of saving. They may be government-sponsored and mandatory, as is Social Security, but the earlier one joins a retirement plan of any type the greater his benefits.

In addition to providing a sense of worth and meaningfulness for the retiree, part-time employment can also provide additional revenue which can supplement the retirement income. Persons receiving Social Security benefits can earn only a certain amount stipulated by federal law. If more than the allowed income is earned, the retiree may lose his Social Security benefits for varying amounts of time. Since Social Security regulations and payments vary for each person and change from year to year, specific figures are not quoted here. The latest information may be obtained by contacting the nearest Social Security office.

Adjusting to the Retirement Income

Not only must the retired couple adjust to newfound leisure time, but their retirement income may necessitate changes or modifications in their living arrangements. The extent of the change depends a great deal on the amount of retirement income the couple has. For those who are not solely dependent on a reduced fixed income, there will probably be no significant change in living patterns. In fact, couples who are in upper income brackets tend to get better housing as they grow older. Families in middle income brackets usually have the finances to remain in essentially the same type of living quarters. It is the poor who are forced into substandard housing in retirement.

Frequently, the retired couple will continue to live in the place they consider home as long as they are able. When this is possible, living adjustments do not need to be made, since friends and neighbors remain the same, and there is no need to worry about facing an unfamiliar environment. Sometimes the couple can rent out part of the house and earn some extra money, which will not affect Social Security benefits.

Sometimes, however, homeowners wish to simplify their living arrangements and responsibilities when they retire. The husband no longer wants to worry about making repairs in the home, cutting the grass, or shoveling the snow. In some cases these responsibilities mean expenditures of money for repairmen and others, which of course deplete fixed-income resources.

What are some of the factors that the couple should consider before moving? The principal ones include climate, recreation, hobby or work opportunities, social groups, transportation, churches or synagogues, hospitals, shopping areas, cost of living, and most of all, personal preferences.

Moving to warmer climates has become increasingly popular in recent years, and retirement villages have sprung up in these areas. Living in a warmer climate helps the clothing budget, since only one weight of clothing is needed. The couple's decision to move may also be influenced by health problems and their desire to get away from winter's toll of upper respiratory infections. Eight chapters of *The Retirement Handbook* by Joseph Buckley are devoted to locations suited to the retired couple. Climatic data are given for selected cities, and there is an in-depth discussion of retirement housing. Villages and apartments designed especially for older Americans are growing at a phenomenal rate. They provide living accommodations with built-in safety features, such as grab bars near the bathtub and toilet, and social and recreational programs. The number of couples living in mobile homes is also increasing. Mobile homeowners may choose their own homesite, and mobile home parks are as diversified as other communities.

When a couple moves from one location to another, there are bound to be adjustments, the nature of these adjustments depending upon the location. If the couple moves from one part of the town to another, the most important things, such as nearness to relatives, friends, and social groups, remain the same. If the couple moves some distance, however, adjustments are more complex. Establishing social contacts, adjusting to a new community, finding the nearest grocery store, looking for a new doctor and dentist—all can be frustrating experiences.

In some situations a couple may find it necessary to move in with their children. The extent to which the retired couple and the children with whom they live have to adjust depends on previously established relationships. Cramped living conditions, young grandchildren underfoot, and constant activity can be difficult for those who look for peace and quiet in the later years.

A sudden permanent move from one area to another is not the best approach. A trial period in the new area is recommended, so that the couple can experiment with the new surroundings before giving up their previous residence. If they find that the new location is not what they thought it to be, they can then return to the familiar place they call home.

Shopping

For those with reduced fixed incomes, shopping for food and clothing may take on new considerations. The couple may tend to avoid high-cost food items and, therefore, reduce proteins by substituting bulk carbohydrates. The couple may justify the lack of protein in the diet on the grounds that decreased physical activity does not warrant the luxury of meat every day. The basic four foods are still needed, however, although not necessarily in the quantities consumed during more active periods of life. Retirees need assistance in learning how to stretch their food dollars and still maintain a balanced diet. Food stamps assist some retired couples in purchasing needed foods. To determine their eligibility, couples must contact the local welfare agency in their community. By prudent planning, careful buying, and effective preparation and storage of food, a couple can be as well nourished on a limited income as on a higher one. Since food plays such an important part in life, one cannot retire from the responsibility of proper eating.

Health Care Costs

The retired couple must also make adjustments and allowances in the budget for increased health care costs. With rising medical and dental rates, families with fixed incomes are particularly hard pressed. Enrollment in some kind of health insurance plan early in married life is an absolute must. If the couple waits until retirement age, they will find the door of insurance companies closed or that they must undergo rigorous physical examinations before a policy will be written. Even if they are successful in obtaining insurance, the premiums will be high in cost.

Government-sponsored health insurance (Medicare) is available to persons age sixty-five and over. Retirees are not automatically enrolled and must apply for the benefits within specified time periods. Participants are charged a modest fee. Details about Medicare can be obtained from local Social Security offices.

The American Association of Retired Persons has health care insurance available to its members and also has a drug service. This mail order service affords considerable savings for those wishing to take advantage of it. The doctor's original prescription is sent to one of the four locations serving the entire country. The prescription is filled and mailed to the retiree. No charge is made for postage, and the patient is billed. Members receive an annual catalog listing nonprescription items. The drug service is especially advantageous for those whose drug bills are high due to long-term illness.

Satisfaction Within the Family

It has been a long time since the husband and wife have spent so much time with one another. With the exception of their honeymoon and vacations, the retired couple have had two separate lives together.

The woman still has many things to keep her occupied around the house. (As always, the washing, ironing, cooking, cleaning still need to be done.) She may tend to overlook her husband's emotional needs. The wife must adjust her life and routines, so that her husband is not merely underfoot around the house. The couple could begin to share some of the household duties—grocery shopping, washing the dishes, spring cleaning. At no other period in their lives does a couple have so much time to enjoy each other's company. These can really be the golden years if the spouses have maintained mutual interests throughout their marriage. Both desperately need to feel needed, worthwhile, and loved, and they can meet these needs for each other if their marriage has been built on a lifetime of loving. It will take time, but new patterns of living will be established now that the tensions and pressures of work have ended. Breakfast can be a leisurely treat with no rush, no bustle, and a second cup of coffee. Hopefully, the couple will begin to reestablish close relationships with each other.

It is important for the retirees to maintain and strengthen ties with their children and to take an interest in the younger family members. Sometimes the retirees may be living in the home of one of their children, which can be a very happy arrangement if there is careful planning. Two cooks in the kitchen can be one too many, but they should be able to agree on a workable schedule that will avoid conflict. The men of the house should also work together to prevent the tensions that could arise.

Grandchildren are a special joy to the older couple. They can spend time with their grandchildren without all the trials and tribulations of child rearing. Live-in grandparents may experience a few problems. They may resent being used as constant live-in baby-sitters, and they may not approve of some newfangled methods of raising children. Grandparents are experts at spoiling grandchildren, and this, too, can be a source of discord in the family. Tact, patience, and communication between retired parents and their children will help to avert some conflicts. Many times both will have to bite their tongues in order to keep peace in the family.

Some retired couples are responsible for the care of an aging parent. They may have this person at home with them or be responsible for maintaining the aged parent in a nursing home. The financial burden and the lack of independence created by this situation can be very trying for the retired couple. If their income is limited, other family members may have to assume some financial responsibility. If there is no other source of income, the retired couple may have to seek help from the local welfare department. This is very difficult for many retired people to do, because they wish to retain their pride and independence and consider public assistance degrading.

When money is no problem, however, the question of independence and freedom still remains. Some retired couples with a dependent parent arrange for the parent to vacation with grandchildren or other relatives so that all may have a change of scene; or the aged person may choose to spend several weeks at a resort for the elderly or a rest home while the children (the retired couple) take a trip. When the aged person is at home and disabled, it may be possible for other family members to stay with great grandmother while the retirees are out of the house.

If contacts with nieces, nephews, cousins, etc., have been emotionally satisfying, they should be maintained. A retired couple's visit to a home-bound niece, who has a houseful of preschool children, can be a treat for all. The young mother is overjoyed to talk to other adults, and the children are delighted with their aunt and uncle. On the other hand, some families have never had relationships that were friendly and satisfying. In this case the retired couple will continue their life-long habit of avoiding the family.

The lives of retired people are like a rich tapestry with many beautiful fibers and colors. Each thread represents an experience of living. This tapestry is not to be hung on a wall and admired, for it is not yet completed. The tapestry is really never finished, for as the last new threads are added, the first ones are pulled out and rewoven into a new tapestry that is a new life.

DEATH

One of the developmental tasks to be accomplished by the aging adult is accepting the reality of death. Many people do not like to talk or think about death; however, during this stage of life one needs to develop a meaningful philosophy toward life and death.[2] Many people will find comfort in their lifelong religious beliefs; others will have to work out their thoughts and attitudes in a different frame of reference.

The husband and wife need to discuss this reality, no matter how painful the subject, because certain realistic plans need to be made in order to prepare for the death of one of them. They should maintain their hospitalization insurance at all costs, for a final illness could be financially disastrous. Both husband and wife should visit their lawyer to have a will drawn or to review and revise their present will if necessary. Any special wishes, such as donation of corneas to eye banks, should be recorded and all legal preparations finalized.

Spouses should know the location of valuable papers and records and the whereabouts of bankbooks, keys to safe-deposit boxes, etc. Funeral arrangements should be discussed, and instructions recorded and placed in a safe location. If burial is desired, a cemetery plot should be purchased and the deed filed in a safe location.

Adjustment to the death of a beloved partner is very difficult, and preparations that may relieve the remaining spouse of unnecessary worry are essential.

Bereavement and Widowhood

The final illness of a husband or wife is a severe emotional strain. Death comes as a final blow, severing the partnership and creating a lonely "oneness." The emotionally exhausted survivor has periods of grief and sorrow and recurrent periods of remorse. It is not unusual for a bereaved person to feel anger toward the person who has gone, a childlike emotion of "Why did you do this to me?" The remaining partner may experience a feeling of relief when a spouse who has suffered through a prolonged terminal illness dies. This relief may turn to feelings of guilt because the surviving spouse feels he should not welcome the death of his partner.

Somehow people recover from the loss of their spouse, but they may never be the same. The loneliness is ever present. In addition to saying "I miss him" or "I miss her," widows and widowers frequently comment on how the deceased partner was taken for granted.

The adjustment to aloneness may involve many changes—a reduction in income, loss of friends, lack of social life, and the assumption of new responsibilities. These changes will be different for the widow than they will be for the widower. Some of the widow's new responsibilities might be automobile maintenance, house repair and upkeep, banking, investments, record keeping, and lawn and garden maintenance. The widower might have to add cooking, laundry, grocery shopping, washing dishes, and sewing to his daily routine. Little things can become major problems. A leaky faucet, for example, can seem like Niagara Falls to a widow who can barely afford the cost of a plumber.

Many widows and widowers think that their feelings of remorse, loneliness, and frustration are abnormal. To the contrary, all bereaved persons experience these feelings. There are many excellent books on the subject of widowhood and widowerhood, and the local library can provide a listing of these. In addition to discussing the normal emotions of a person in grief, these books give examples of how to manage the day-to-day routine of new responsibilities and problems.

The surviving partner is advised to postpone any major decisions until a year after the death of the spouse. At this time situations will be viewed more realistically than during the period of acute grief.

The adjustment to living alone is very difficult, and maintaining social contacts requires a conscious effort on the part of the lonely spouse. With support from friends and relatives and a continuing of one's social, religious, and community activities, the widow or widower will be able to maintain a meaningful life.

Remarriage

Most often it is the woman who is widowed, since statistics reveal that women tend to have a longer life span than men. Approximately 50 percent of the women and 20 percent of the men age sixty-five have lost their spouses. Studies are now being made to determine the percentage of remarriages after the age of sixty-five.

American society has, in the past, frowned on the very idea of remarriage or marriage among its older citizens. In effect, this attitude implies that with increasing chronological age comes a decreased need for love, sex, affection, and companionship. How far from the truth this assumption is. These emotional and social needs are not dependent on the age of an individual but are basic human needs for everyone regardless of age. Loneliness and isolation from social activities once enjoyed with the spouse are realities of life for the widowed.

Men tend to remarry more frequently than women, and the new bride is usually considerably younger than the man. Women are less likely to remarry for a variety of reasons. One is the competition with much younger women; another is that they outnumber the men. Furthermore, the widow's Social Security benefits will cease upon remarriage if they are based on her first husband's earnings.

The number of marriages among those sixty-five and over seems to be increasing. The prime motivation for remarriage is the fulfillment of those needs previously mentioned. Other factors, not usually expressed by the individual anticipating remarriage, may be (1) a desire to escape from a stressful situation, perhaps being merely tolerated while residing at the home of a son or daughter, (2) a desire for one's own home, and (3) an enhancing of one's social status by marrying someone of a higher financial and social level. These reasons are not of course those that ensure a successful retirement marriage or remarriage. Factors that contribute to the success of the marriage include the couple's ability to adjust to each other and to new situations, good health, and a lack of major disabilities.

Frequently, the bride and groom have known each other for many years as family friends or have been related by the previous marriage. In this case the future partner will be accepted by family and friends, which makes adjustment to the marriage much easier.

Senior citizens' clubs, church groups, and community activities all provide opportunities for older Americans to meet and socialize. Although the purpose of these activities is not to produce retirement romances, this can be a bonus outcome of membership.

The average Social Security payment for a retired couple in 1971 was $218 per month or $2,616 per year. Since the widow who remarries loses Social Security benefits derived from her first husband's employment, the widow may accept friendship and companionship rather than enter into marriage. Some couples share apartments and living expenses in an effort to stretch limited incomes, thus obtaining companionship without losing their Social Security.

In summary, a good second marriage can make the remaining years enjoyable and retirement more successful. As one man explained, "I have more time to enjoy what I have. I don't have more money, perhaps less, but I now get more kick out of life. When you are on the sidelines with a partner, you can enjoy the game more."[3]

THE SINGLE ADULT

Although the developmental tasks of the single adult do not differ from those of the married person, the unmarried retiree must accomplish these tasks without the support of a spouse. If gainful employment has been the person's major source of social and emotional satisfaction, retirement will create a severe void, necessitating a greater social adjustment than is necessary for a married person. The single adult appears to be better equipped to cope with the financial aspects of retirement, however, and since he has been functioning independently for most of his adult life, he does not experience the "lonely oneness" of bereavement.

STUDY QUESTIONS AND PROBLEMS

1. Mrs. Lewis has been very lonely since the death of her husband a year ago. They had enjoyed his five years of retirement. Mrs. Lewis would like to join a club of retired people so that she can make some new friends and have someplace to go. How would she go about finding such a club and becoming a member?
2. Does your community have a volunteer service bureau? Where is it located? If not, what other resources are available to retired persons who wish to become volunteer workers?
3. Read the help wanted ads in your local newspaper and clip any that could be filled by a retired person. Bring these ads to class and discuss the availability of part-time jobs for older adults.
4. Prepare a list of the adult education programs in your community.
5. How would an aged couple go about retaining the services of a lawyer for the preparation of a will? What are the usual fees for this type of service?
6. Visit your local public library and prepare a list of books and pamphlets written to aid the widow or widower in his adjustment.

BIBLIOGRAPHY

Buckley, Joseph C. *The Retirement Handbook.* 3rd ed. New York: Harper & Row, 1967.

Duvall, Evelyn. *Family Development.* 4th ed. Philadelphia: J. B. Lippincott, 1971.

Farr, William. "The Law and Your Retirement." *Modern Maturity.* February-March 1970.

Genn, Lillian G. "Boom in Retirement Marriage." *Modern Maturity.* February-March 1970.

Havighurst, R. J. *Human Development and Education.* New York: Longmans, Green, 1953.

"Institute of Lifetime Learning." *Modern Maturity.* February-March 1970.

Lidz, Theodore. *The Person, His Development Throughout the Life Cycle.* New York: Basic Books, 1968.

"Mature Temps." *Modern Maturity.* August-September 1970.

Mitchell, H. S.; Rynbergen, H. J.; Anderson, L.; and Dibble, M. V. *Cooper's Nutrition in Health and Disease.* 15th ed. Philadelphia: J. B. Lippincott, 1968.

U.S., Administration on Aging, *Are You Planning on Living the Rest of Your Life?* AOA Washington, D.C.: Department of Health, Education, and Welfare, Publication No. 803. U.S. Government Printing Office, 1964.

U.S., Department of Health, Education, and Welfare, *Working with Older People—A Guide to Practice,* vol. 2, *Biological, Psychological and Sociological Aspects of Aging.* Washington, D.C.: U.S. Government Printing Office, 1970.

U.S., Department of Health, Education, and Welfare, *Working with Older People—A Guide to Practice,* vol. 3, *The Aging Person: Needs and Services.* Washington, D.C.: U.S. Government Printing Office, 1970.

NOTES

1. Evelyn Duvall, *Family Development,* 4th ed. (Philadelphia: J. B. Lippincott, 1971).
2. Duvall, *Family Development,* p. 439.
3. Lillian Genn, "Boom in Retirement Marriage," *Modern Maturity.* February-March 1970, p. 14.

3

The Community and the Older Adult

In the preceding chapter the role of the aging person in a youth-oriented culture was discussed, and the contributions that the older citizen can make to the community were emphasized. While the retiree has much to offer to the community, so, too, the community has much to offer the aging person.

Almost every community in the United States can boast of at least one senior citizens' club. Such clubs are usually sponsored by a community group, which may or may not be the local recreation department. The local government usually pays for the rental and maintenance of meeting places for these groups.

PUBLIC HOUSING

Throughout the United States municipalities have built and maintained housing for senior citizens. Such housing is designed to meet the needs of these people and provides special safety features to prevent accidents. These buildings usually have ramps, walkways, and elevators that give the handicapped person access to the building. The major benefit in public housing is the rent scale, which remains at a fairly constant and inexpensive level. Furthermore, the residents need not be concerned with interior or exterior maintenance of their dwellings. In very large cities the housing for senior citizens may have a senior citizens' club, social service agency, medical clinic, and branch library located within the complex of buildings. In many communities elaborate residences have been built for elderly citizens as a part of urban renewal projects—funded largely by the federal government. When a senior citizens' residence is located in an urban area, there are usually problems, such as transportation to and from the supermarket, the church or synagogue, the doctor's office, etc. Although there may be easy access to public transportation, it is difficult for elderly people to get on and off a bus and to carry two grocery bags without falling or dropping the food. When the construction of housing for the elderly is being planned, there should always be a representative from this group of citizens, who best know their own needs, wants, and problems.

All public housing is administered by a local housing authority. It is the business of this agency to provide decent, safe, and sanitary housing for low-income families at rents they can afford. The United States Department of Housing and Urban Development (HUD) provides financial, technical, and administrative assistance for publicly controlled units specifically designed for elderly tenants. Interestingly, the 1970 Housing Act provides funds for the financing of a group dining room in publicly built housing for senior citizens.

COMMUNITY HEALTH PROGRAMS

In many communities there are no special health programs for the aged, and the retired person must solve his health problems alone. The ways in which he can meet his health needs have been discussed earlier. However, local agencies, such as county cancer societies and county heart associations, may conduct diagnostic detection surveys at senior citizens' centers. Very few hospitals have clinics designed specifically for the area of geriatrics, and very few physicians (and other health professionals) feel comfortable working in this field of medicine. In large cities, however, where senior citizen housing is in a complex of several high-rise buildings, the local health department may run specialized clinics for the aged.

MEALS ON WHEELS AND OTHER FOOD PROGRAMS

The nutritional needs of the elderly person may be met by the community in a variety of ways. Many aging persons are able to remain in their own homes but are unable to do any food shopping and preparation. Meals on Wheels is a project that provides one or two meals a day for senior citizens. The food is prepared in a central location—hospital kitchen, visiting nurse association, nursing home, local school, church, etc.—and delivered by truck to the elderly client. One meal may be hot and one cold (sandwich, fruit, and milk). All menus provide for adequate nutrition and any special dietary requirements. The fee for this service is based on the client's ability to pay, or a sliding scale. Volunteers from the community take the food from the truck and deliver it to the senior citizen. If the aged person is ill or requests some other type of service, the volunteer reports this to the Meals on Wheels director, who makes the proper referral. In addition to meeting the nutritional needs of the aged, this program may also help to meet their social needs. Many have no visitors other than the Meals on Wheels volunteers, who may come daily or five times a week. The volunteer servers often become good friends with their clients.

Other community programs may include walk-in feeding programs, in which one, two, or three meals may be obtained at a senior citizens' meal center. These meals are usually inexpensive and, again, meet both nutritional and social needs.

The retired couple or individual with a low fixed income may qualify for assistance with his grocery bills under the federal Food Stamp Plan. After purchasing these stamps, he can use the coupons as food money, which has a higher value than the original investment. Food stamps can be used to buy any kind of *food* at the grocery store. Thus, the food stamp program increases the purchasing power of persons with limited financial resources. Information concerning food stamps can be obtained from the local welfare agency or food stamp program office.

THE ADMINISTRATION ON AGING

The Administration on Aging (AOA) is one of the units of the Welfare Administration of the Department of Health, Education, and Welfare (HEW). It is the national clearing house for information for aging Americans from the Bureau of Family Services, the Office of Education, and the Housing and Home Finance Agency. The Administration on Aging works with state and local agencies (offices on aging) in their efforts to bring essential services to the elderly. In addition, the administration publishes the monthly news magazine *Aging* as well as other printed materials about the elderly population, housing, and grant programs. More information about the Administration on Aging may be obtained by writing the AOA, Social Security Administration, Department of Health, Education, and Welfare, Washington, D.C.

SOCIAL SECURITY

The Social Security legislation provides four different kinds of benefits. These are (1) retirement benefits, (2) survivors' benefits to widows, widowers, children, and dependent parents, (3) death benefits to the surviving spouse, and (4) disability benefits.

As discussed in Chapter 2, the employee and his employer make Social Security payments to the federal government. This money is placed in a special fund and is withdrawn when the worker's earnings stop due to retirement, death, or disability. The amount of money received from Social Security depends on the length of time the person has been enrolled in the program and the amount of salary on which the payments were based. Any questions concerning Social Security should be referred to a district office of this agency. This office should be consulted when (1) a worker in the family dies, (2) one becomes disabled, (3) retirement age (minimum age sixty-two) approaches, and (4) one reaches age seventy-two. (At seventy-two a person may work full time and collect full benefits.) Certain requirements must be met in order for survivors' benefits to be collected; therefore the Social Security office should be contacted. Lump-sum death benefits are paid to the widow or widower, which helps to pay the funeral costs. If there is no surviving spouse, this money goes to the person who paid the funeral director.

MEDICARE

Medicare is a federally sponsored hospital and medical insurance plan under the Social Security law and has been available since 1966. It is financed by Social Security payments, and almost everyone over the age of sixty-five is eligible to enroll in this insurance plan. However, the retiree is not automatically enrolled at the age of sixty-five. There are specific times when one can enroll in this insurance plan, and the Social Security office should be contacted regarding enrollment before the person reaches his sixty-fifth birthday. Detailed information concerning Medicare may be obtained from all local district offices.

Medicare is made up of two kinds of insurance coverage. Part A provides basic protection against costs of inpatient hospital care, post-hospital extended care, and post-hospital home health care. This portion is financed mainly through Social Security monies. Part B is a voluntary medical insurance plan and provides protection against costs of physicians' services, medical service and supplies, home health care, outpatient services, and other types of service. The enrollee pays one-half of a small monthly premium for this insurance, and the federal government pays the other half. In 1971 20.6 million people were enrolled in the Medicare hospital plan, and 19.7 million were signed up for voluntary medical insurance. Nearly 10 percent of all the people in the United States are protected by Medicare.

In addition to providing protection against the financial ravages of illness, the Medicare legislation sets high standards for patient care. For example, nursing homes that treat Medicare enrollees are required to have twenty-four-hour-a-day nursing service with at least one full-time registered nurse and a doctor to handle emergencies. Other Medicare regulations concern the nursing home's medical and nursing policies, special procedures, and methods for handling and dispensing drugs.

MEDICAID

As the name implies, Medicaid, or Medical Assistance Program, provides medical assistance for certain kinds of needy people. These include those over sixty-five, the blind, and members of families with dependent children. Medicaid is administered by state governments according to federal guidelines. In some states the Medical Assistance Program covers *only* people who are eligible for public assistance (welfare). In other states the determination for eligibility may be slightly less stringent. Applicants for Medicaid should contact their local welfare or public assistance office.

THE OLDER AMERICANS ACT

The Older Americans Act was enacted in 1965 and extended in 1967. The most recent legislation proposes a total of $257 million to be spent on the aging population in 1973. Title I of the act contains a bill of rights for older Americans, which includes:

adequate income

housing to meet special needs

restorative services in institutions caring for the aged

employment opportunities

retirement with dignity and honor plus recognition of contributions to the economy during working years

opportunity to pursue meaningful activities

coordinated and efficient community services

immediate benefits from pertinent research findings that may improve health and happiness

opportunity for the individual to take the initiative in planning and managing his own life and future

The Older Americans Act established the Administration on Aging and the state offices on aging. The law and the agencies created by it have made the nation more aware of the older American and his problems. Many programs initiated for the aged have brought them together in working organizations that seek community support for their programs.

Senior power—a true political force—cannot be denied. In some states senior citizens have been effective in gaining special real estate tax deductions for themselves. Older Americans will continue to be more vocal and forceful with legislators at all levels.

GREEN THUMB/GREEN LIGHT PROJECT

The Green Thumb/Green Light Project is designed to meet the needs of the aged poor living in rural areas. It is under the jurisdiction of the Department of Labor and is sponsored by the National Farmers Union. Retired men may be paid up to $1,600 yearly for work on beautification projects, such as highway roadside improvement and historical restoration. (See Figure 3-1.) Women may participate (Green Light) and be paid as teachers' aides and workers in school kitchens.

VOLUNTEER FRIENDLY VISITOR SERVICE

Many communities and states have instituted a volunteer program in which mature men and women visit the homebound on a regular basis. These programs, sponsored and supervised by a local community agency, are designed to bring friendship with understanding to the chronically ill and socially isolated persons in need of companionship. Following a short

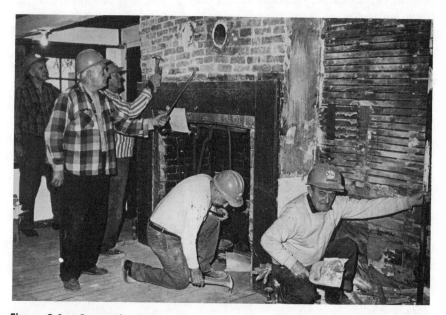

Figure 3-1: Green Thumbers work on the restoration of an historical site. *(N.J. Farmers Union, Green Thumb Project)*

training course and orientation, the volunteer makes weekly home visits during which he socializes with the homebound person and may also write letters for him, read aloud to him, play cards and games, encourage the initiation of simple handicrafts, and run errands such as shopping (with the agency's approval). This service not only provides a social contact for the homebound but also allows his already overburdened family members some precious free time away from constant responsibilities. Senior citizens who are in good health may also become a part of this volunteer social service, thereby meeting the needs of the community and their own age group.

The federal government, as well as state and local governments, has been active in *beginning* to meet the needs of the aging population. However, the White House Conference on Aging held in November of 1971 suggested many areas for future efforts on behalf of the elderly citizen. Many of the recommendations concern areas in which the government is already active—housing, nutrition, health, and economy. The delegates indicated a need for increased and renewed work in these areas and a special effort toward the solution of the pressing problems of the aged.

STUDY QUESTIONS AND PROBLEMS

1. How has your community become involved with the institutionalized aged? Does your community provide services such as mobile voter registration, absentee ballots, transportation service to and from the polls, and mobile library services?
2. Where are your state and local offices on aging located? What services do they provide?
3. Visit the district Social Security office and determine the minimum and maximum retirement benefits paid to single and married retirees.

BIBLIOGRAPHY

A Community Guide: Housing New Jersey's Elderly. State of New Jersey, Office on Aging: Trenton, N.J., 1970.
Ellenbogen, Gladys. *Aging in New Jersey: An Economic Analysis*. Montclair, N.J.: Montclair State College, 1971.
Laas, William. *Helpful Hints on Managing Your Money for Retirement*. New York: Popular Library, 1970.
1971 White House Conference on Aging. A Report to the Delegates from the Conference Sections and Special Concerns Sessions. Washington, D.C.: U.S. Government Printing Office, 1971.
Statistical Abstract of the United States, 1972. U.S. Government Printing Office, Washington, D.C.: 1972.
Steele, Harold, and Crow, Charles. *How to Deal with Aging and the Elderly*. Huntsville, Ala.: The Strode Publishers, 1970.
Townsend, Claire. *Old Age: The Last Segregation*. New York: Grossman Publishers, 1971.

U.S., Department of Health, Education, and Welfare, Medical Services Administration, Social and Rehabilitation Service, *Medicaid and Medicare—Which is Which?* Washington, D.C.: U.S. Government Printing Office, 1971.

U.S., Department of Health, Education, and Welfare, Social Security Administration. *Medicare Benefits in an Extended Care Facility.* DHEW Publishing No. (SSA) 72-10041, Washington, D.C.: U.S. Government Printing Office, 1971.

U.S., Department of Health, Education, and Welfare, Social Security Administration, *Your Medicare Handbook.* Washington, D.C.: U.S. Government Printing Office, 1972.

U.S., Department of Health, Education, and Welfare, Social Security Administration, *Social Security Benefits—How You Earn Them—How to Estimate the Amount.* DHEW Publishing No. (SSA) 72-10047, Washington, D.C.: U.S. Government Printing Office, 1971.

U.S., Department of Health, Education, and Welfare, Social Security Administration, *Your Social Security.* DHEW Publishing No. (SSA) 72-10035, U.S. Government Printing Office, Washington, D.C.: 1972.

West, Howard. "Five Years of Medicare—A Statistical Review." *Social Security Bulletin,* December, 1971.

4

The Normal Aging Process and How to Cope with It

The process of aging begins at birth and is most rapid in infancy, becoming progressively slower in childhood and maturity, and affecting different tissues at different rates.[1] The physiological changes commonly associated with aging, then, started many, many years prior to the outward appearances we link with "growing old." It is one's successful adjustment to these changes in body structure and function that accounts for the phrase "healthy old age."

SKELETOMUSCULAR CHANGES

The most obvious change in the skeletomuscular system is the shortened stature of the elderly. This is due to a shortening of the spinal column. X-ray studies of the elderly reveal a narrowing of the vertebral discs caused by osteoporosis, a decrease in bone mass, or density, without any change in its chemistry. This condition is almost universally found in elderly women.[2] Thus the aged person has a shortened trunk with relatively long extremities.

The overall shortening of the vertebral column produces kyphosis of the upper thoracic spine (Dowager's hump or humpback). This curvature causes the person's head to be tilted backward, since there are also changes in the bony structure of the neck. In addition to postural changes produced by osteoporosis, the bones become increasingly brittle and subject to fractures. This is especially true of the long bones.

There are many theories about the cause of osteoporosis in the aged,

34

including lack of activity throughout the person's life span, lack of adequate calcium intake during adulthood, inability of the body to utilize calcium, and hormonal changes associated with the menopause and the aging process.

Some joints may have degenerative changes that produce a decrease in the range of motion, while other joints may be more mobile due to stretching of the ligaments. In general, there is some deterioration in muscle control, and the older person will complain about his lack of strength and how quickly he tires.

The degenerative changes in the skeletomuscular system cannot be reversed, but the elderly individual can take measures that will enable him to live with these limitations. It is important that he maintain good posture and proper body alignment. A lifetime of good posture may be a factor in preventing or decreasing degenerative curvatures of the spine. Proper shoes and a broad base of support are prerequisites for a straight stance. Tennis shoes and sandals provide inadequate support for aging feet and should not be used as a substitute for shoes.

Many older persons complain that if they sit too long their joints become stiff and they have difficulty walking and moving. This should be reason enough for the aged to keep active. The daily routine should include a regular program of moderate exercise that will make use of all joints and most muscles. One of the least expensive and most efficient activities is walking. Ideally, this activity will be the continuance of a lifetime habit. If a new type of exercise is adopted, the family physician should be consulted before it is instituted. Programs of physical fitness are offered in many communities by senior citizens' clubs and YMCAs or YMHAs. Many retired men and women continue to bowl, golf, fish, bicycle, but at a more leisurely pace than before.

The elderly person must remember that he will tire more easily than he did in the past, and he should not be discouraged by this. The purpose of exercise and activity is not exhaustion, but to keep the machinery functioning as smoothly as possible. When the signs of tiring begin to appear, the activity should be stopped, and the older person should rest. It is far better to play nine holes of golf, bowl two games, walk the dog three blocks and feel refreshed than to overdo the activity and become completely fatigued.

Caution must be an essential part of any activity, since even a slight fall can result in a serious bone fracture. The elderly must be constantly alert to hazards that might cause an accident. Little things like unmended shoes, floppy slippers, and trailing shoelaces could result in a nasty fall.

Other dangerous items are slippery throw rugs, dangling electric and tele-phone cords, open drawers, poorly lit stairways, and pets underfoot.

There are safety items that should be added to the older person's living quarters to ease mobility and prevent accidents. Examples are grab bars adjacent to tubs, showers, and toilets; sturdy handrailings on stair-ways; adequate lighting at both the top and the bottom of steps; and non-slip mats or strips in showers, tubs, and in front of the kitchen sink. Good housekeeping can also reduce the possibility of accidents. Spilled liquids should be removed from floors; ice and snow should be removed from walks and steps. The elderly person should not shovel snow, however. This activity is much too strenuous. Snow- and ice-melting chemicals should be applied, a snow shoveler hired, or a neighbor or relative asked to assume this responsibility.

Although the role of calcium in preventing osteoporosis has not been definitely determined, proper diet, including recommended minimum daily amounts of vitamins, minerals, and other nutrients, is encouraged. Milk is a good source of calcium, and the older person should consume at least a pint of milk daily. This may be used in cream soups, desserts, or as a refreshing drink. Nonfat dry milk is an inexpensive source of calcium and can be used in cooking.

Since elderly women have a high incidence of osteoporosis and re-sultant fractures, many researchers are looking into the effects of the menopause on the skeletal system. The administration of female hormones to postmenopausal patients appears to ward off the development or pro-gression of osteoporosis. Unfortunately, these hormones have many un-desirable side effects. Research has not determined their applicability for broad use in the prevention and treatment of osteoporosis.

The degenerative changes in the skeletomuscular system are progres-sive, but they need not be debilitating. With some modification in ways of living, the elderly person should be able to enjoy his retirement without undergoing any severe limitations of movement and activity.

CIRCULATORY-RESPIRATORY CHANGES

We tend to think of the circulatory and respiratory systems as those that present the most problems. Cardiovascular diseases cause more deaths annually in the United States than all other diseases combined. Because of this fact, it is difficult to see that some normal processes of aging affect this system and do not involve disease but rather must be known and coped with by the older person. A look at these changes will provide clues to the adjustments in daily living that the elderly must make.

A decrease in the metabolic rate associated with decreased production of body heat results in a lowering of body temperature. Although the normal range of body temperature for the healthy adult is 97° F. to 99°F., there is a greater variation in range for the healthy aged. It is possible, then, for an elderly person who has an upper respiratory infection to have a temperature of 98.6°F. and have it represent a fever. The pulse and respiration of the elderly also show wide variations. Unless the individual's normal temperature, pulse, and respiration are known, it is difficult to ascertain deviations from normal solely by measuring vital signs. The early morning temperature may be 95°F. The nurse must be sure to shake the thermometer down far enough to obtain an accurate reading.

Blood pressure determinations show an increase in both the systolic and the diastolic pressure. This phenomenon is not to be confused with hypertension in which the significant increase is found in the diastolic pressure. It is rare for the healthy person to be concerned with his vital signs. We don't often hear of someone complaining of an increased systolic pressure! It is not uncommon, however, for the elderly to complain about being cold, which is a symptom of the aging process that is related to changes within the circulatory system. With the diminished supply of blood to the coronary arteries, the heart is not as effective in its pumping action, and the extremities do not receive the amount of blood they did in the past. Decrease in physical activity, a lower metabolic rate, and the high incidence of arteriosclerotic vessels all contribute to this phenomenon of the aging process. The most effective way for the older person to relieve this symptom is to wear warmer clothing. Emphasis should be placed on warmth, not weight. In this day of synthetic fibers, it is easy to find clothing that is both warm and lightweight. A word of caution should be given to the older adult: Avoid the use of hot-water bottles and other forms of dry or moist heat. The extremities, while cold, may also be insensitive to extreme heat. Severe burns have occurred in persons who have used a hot-water bottle that was too hot.

The power of the heart is reduced, and more energy is expended in the process of contracting the heart muscle. When sudden increased stress is placed on the heart, the person finds it more difficult to adjust. For instance, the woman who at one time was able to vacuum the floor vigorously without stopping for a half hour finds that now she must stop frequently to rest.

As the body ages, the elasticity of the blood vessels diminishes. It is believed that the increase in calcium deposits in the vessels is a factor contributing to this loss of elasticity. Any clothing that tends to reduce an already restricted blood supply to the extremities should be eliminated from the wardrobe. Serious offenders are round garters or elastic rubber bands elderly women depend on to hold up their stockings. Clothing should be of the comfortable, nonconstricting type.

Standing for long periods of time causes the pooling of blood in the extremities. As a result, there is a decrease in blood supply to the brain and dizziness occurs. This is the time when accidents are likely to happen. Sudden changes in position may also create temporary circulatory problems.

Because of these physiological changes, the elderly person should plan a balance of activity and rest so that the circulatory system will be able to accommodate itself to the work load.

The majority of older persons demonstrate some degree of anemia, in which the hemoglobin levels are reduced. Although this is more often the case with women than with men, the fact emphasizes the need for protein and other foods high in iron content.

Changes in the musculoskeletal system also affect the functioning of the respiratory system. Kyphosis and osteoporosis reduce the size of the chest wall, and the reduced chest size creates a rigidity not previously in evidence. As with the circulatory system, there is a decrease in the elasticity of the tracheobronchial tree. The alveoli decrease in number and increase in size, and the bronchioles become dilated. Even with these changes the total lung capacity is not altered drastically.

There is, however, a decreased capacity to cough effectively, which is due to the reduced strength of the muscles used in expiration as well as to a rigid chest wall. Although older adults tend to have a high incidence of morning cough, the ability to adequately eliminate mucous secretions is diminished. A contributing factor is also the decreased ciliary activity of the bronchial lining. The elderly, therefore, are more susceptible to infections of the respiratory system and should be careful to avoid situations that would expose them to infections of this nature.

Dyspnea upon increased activity again emphasizes the need for the older person to space those activities that put an increased load on the cardiopulmonary system.

The changes that take place in the circulatory-respiratory systems of the older adult are not necessarily linked with a disease process. The nurse must be knowledgeable about these changes in order to assist the elderly in making those adjustments in their daily activities necessary to accommodate such normal physiological changes.

DIGESTIVE SYSTEM CHANGES

Many elderly people complain that they no longer enjoy eating; food just doesn't taste the way it used to. Their observations are accurate, for a decreased sense of taste is a part of the aging process. This change is brought about by a reduction in the number of taste buds and a decrease in the sense of smell.

Furthermore, the aged may find chewing difficult because they have teeth missing, ill-fitting dentures, or no teeth at all. Teeth are lost for a variety of reasons, ranging from tooth decay to gum and tooth changes produced by the aging process. Unfortunately for those on a limited or fixed income, dental care is a costly investment and older people may choose to go toothless rather than spend their savings for dentures.

Certainly, eating is no pleasure when one is unable to chew his food properly. Anyone who cannot chew easily will eat soft foods and avoid meats, some fruits, and many vegetables. This, of course, will affect his nutrition. In addition, a lack of roughage in the diet and the slowed peristalsis of the digestive tract can produce constipation.

Older adults need the basic four food groups, and their need for nutrients remains essentially unchanged. Many nutritionists feel that fewer calories are needed. The elderly tend to consume large quantities of carbohydrates, which yield many calories but are low in other nutrients. This is because carbohydrates are inexpensive, generally easy to prepare and serve, and satisfy the sweet tooth that appears in old age.

The older person should be urged to seek dental care. Dental clinics may be found in many communities, and dental schools can also provide this type of care at a low cost. If dental work cannot be done, some modifications in the texture of the diet are advised. A food chopper or a blender can be used to prepare foods that are easy to eat. Eggs, ground chuck, and liver are examples of economical, high-protein foods that can be eaten without chewing difficulties. Fruit juices and blended or chopped vegetables can be included in the diet. The importance of milk has been stressed earlier, and all menus should incorporate this food.

Constipation can be prevented by including roughage and adequate amounts of fluid in the diet. Fresh fruits and vegetables can be cut into tiny pieces and served as a salad. Six to eight glasses of fluid should be consumed daily. This may be water, juice, milk, coffee, tea, or boullion. Carbonated beverages are high in caloric content and provide little nutritional value, and thus should be used sparingly.

Indigestion and heartburn are common complaints of the elderly. Very often a review of the diet will reveal that they consume large quantities of fried or highly seasoned foods, which are difficult for most people to digest. These types of foods should be avoided and other methods of cooking employed. Braising, broiling, roasting, and boiling are good methods of preparing foods. Subtle flavoring with herbs may be substituted for spicy seasoning.

The aged palate needs to be tempted by attractive food. Small portions should be served so that the individual is not overwhelmed by the size of the meal. A variety of textures and colors combined with simple cooking techniques, will stimulate the older appetite. A glass of beer, wine, or other favorite alcoholic beverage before dinner may be just the thing to sharpen the appetite and make mealtime more pleasurable.

The digestive system is truly remarkable in its ability to adjust to the changes caused by aging. There is a decrease in the quantity of almost all digestive enzymes (ptyalin, pepsin, trypsin, amylase, and lipase), but even so, the digestive functioning is not impaired. Some changes in liver structure and function do occur, but this organ continues to perform within normal ranges. Absorption of food does not seem to be affected by the aging process.

Elderly people, then, experience discomforts of heartburn, gas, indigestion, and constipation. These problems arise largely from the digestive changes caused by the aging process and by dietary factors. If these symptoms occur regularly and cause severe distress, a physician should be consulted because the threat of cancer is a reality. Many aged persons are convinced that they have cancer of the digestive system, and the nurse should encourage them to discuss this fear with a doctor. Fear of cancer is a terrible worry to live with, and the family doctor will be able to make a diagnosis that will relieve this emotional burden. In most cases dietary changes and moderation will solve the problem. If there are no disease processes present, there is no reason why the aged cannot enjoy eating and stay fit.

GENITOURINARY SYSTEM CHANGES

The arteriosclerotic process also affects the urinary system, particularly the renal arteries supplying the kidney. With the decrease in blood flow to the kidney, there is also a decrease in renal functioning. The number of functioning nephrons is reduced, which also diminishes the filtering ability of the kidney. Despite these changes, however, the kidney continues to function within normal limits.

The bladder may also show the effects of aging. The bladder's capacity to hold urine may be reduced, and as a result, the older person may complain of leaking, which may indicate that the bladder is filled to beyond capacity. Another indication that the bladder is so filled can be the immediate and urgent signal to urinate. In younger adults the desire to void is relayed from the bladder to the brain when the bladder is one-half full. In the aged, however, the awareness is delayed until perhaps the limit of bladder capacity is reached.

Not only is the bladder's capacity to hold urine diminished, but there may also be problems associated with its ability to empty properly. Some urine, known as residual urine, may remain in the bladder immediately after voiding.

With the bladder's reduced capacity comes the need for arising during the night to void. Nocturnal frequency can cause the elderly to make several trips to the bathroom, an annoyance but not necessarily associated with any disease process. One suggestion for coping with this might be to restrict fluid intake after the evening meal. The total normal daily intake of fluid, however, should not be reduced. Those beverages that stimulate voiding, such as coffee and drinks containing alcohol, should be avoided during the course of the evening. At least three or four hours should elapse between the evening meal and bedtime. If the person retires shortly after eating, there is more likelihood of his having to urinate during the night. Foods high in salt content and highly spiced foods should not be included in the last meal of the day.

Because accidents could occur during the nighttime trip to the bathroom, night lights in the bedroom, hall, and bathroom may be indicated. Free, uncluttered passageways to the bathroom are also important, and the elderly person's bedroom should be as near to the bathroom as possible. Another solution would be the use of a commode in the bedroom.

When complaints of frequency and urgency are prevalent in older women, they may be caused by weakness of the sphincter of the urethra. This condition is more noticeable in colder weather.

Changes also take place in the reproductive system of the male. Usually, the size of the prostate gland increases, and sclerotic changes take place in this organ. When the prostate enlarges to the point of constricting the neck of the bladder, urinary symptoms occur.

The ability of the testes to manufacture sperm can remain a function well into the advanced age of the man. In the woman, however, the ovaries atrophy following the menopause, and the activity of producing ova is no longer a function. Because of the change in ovarian hormones during the menopause, the uterus begins to shrink in size, with fibrous tissue replacing some of the myometrium, and the endometrium thins out.

The external genital organs also undergo changes, which become obvious to the older woman. Breast changes resulting from the lack of ovarian hormones are sometimes distressing to the woman. The breasts begin to flatten and sag due to the atrophy of breast tissue. Money spent on creams and ointments to rejuvenate the breasts is money spent unwisely, for these changes are irreversible. The need for continued support for the breasts is indicated, particularly for women with pendulous breasts. Care should be taken to ensure that brassieres fit properly and provide the support needed. The older woman should be encouraged to continue self-examination of the breasts every month with the understanding that this will not take the place of the semiannual examination by her physician.

The fatty tissue of the external genitalia is also reduced, and the mucous membrane lining the vagina flattens, resulting in a reduced quantity of mucous secretion. Because of this, there is an increased tendency toward vaginal inflammation and infection. Itching and discharge are symptoms of senile vaginitis. Pelvic examination with Pap smear should be performed to rule out the possibility of other causes for these symptoms. The older woman should have a pelvic examination at least once yearly; many physicians recommend semiannual exams as a precautionary measure.

Itching associated with the dryness of the genitalia may be an annoying symptom that the older person is reluctant to report to the physician. Very often hot tub baths are a predisposing factor in this condition.

Painful intercourse may occur due to the lack of natural lubrication. Artificial lubrication of the external genitalia with water-soluble lubricating jelly prior to intercourse will help to alleviate this problem. Until recently taboos on discussing sex activities produced the stereotype of the elderly as having no sexual interest, much less any activity in this area. Since we have become more open in discussing sex as a natural part of one's life, studies have verified that "sex after sixty" is not a myth after all! According to Masters and Johnson,

> *There is every reason to believe that maintained regularity of sexual expression coupled with adequate physical well-being and mental health orientation to the aging process will combine to provide a sexually stimulative climate within a marriage. This climate will, in turn, improve sexual tension and provide a capacity for sexual performance that frequently may extend to and beyond the 80-year age level.*[3]

The normally functioning genitourinary system causes relatively few problems for the aged. Those that do occur may be annoying but do not prevent normal activities. Because of the possibilities of disease conditions, the nurse should encourage the aged to have annual or semiannual physical examinations.

ENDOCRINE SYSTEM CHANGES

The major changes in the endocrine system—that of ovarian decline—occurs during the middle years of the woman's life. Research has documented few other changes, and little is known about the effects of the aging process on the ductless glands.

Decrease in hormone production does not appear to affect body structure and function. Altered glucose tolerance tests indicate a change in insulin production or effectiveness, but the evidence is not conclusive. Many persons are diagnosed as pre-diabetics during this period of life, and the elderly, therefore, should be encouraged to participate in free community diabetes screening programs and to watch for the symptoms of this disease condition.

INTEGUMENTARY SYSTEM CHANGES

Throughout the integumentary system there is a change in the distribution of subcutaneous fat. This tissue is lost from the face, arms, and legs and is deposited over the hips and abdomen. The process does not occur on one's sixty-fifth birthday but is an ongoing change that accelerates during the later years. The loss of subcutaneous fat from the arms and legs causes the aged to be especially sensitive to low temperatures. Measures that will aid the elderly in coping with this problem have been discussed earlier.

The fatty tissue enveloping the breasts is reduced, and the glandular tissue in this area atrophy, causing the breasts of elderly women to sag or become smaller. For women who are overly concerned about these changes, a good brassiere can restore youthful appearance. A properly fitted foundation can provide abdominal support and aid in maintaining good posture.

Women with large, pendulous breasts may experience extreme discomfort from skin irritation and chafing in this area. Caked and dry talcum powder, bra bands that are too tight, and cups that do not provide proper support further increase the problem. Daily washing, dusting the area with cornstarch, and suitable undergarments can relieve the discomfort.

Certain bony prominences become more obvious due to the decrease of fatty tissue. Thus, well-fitting clothes should be selected. If the collar bones are especially pronounced, the older person does not have to bring attention to the area by wearing a low-cut neckline. Long sleeves will hide bony elbows and thin forearms as well as provide protection from cold.

The aged skin is very dry and thin, and for this reason daily bathing should be avoided. Certainly, the elderly should wash their skin, but daily tub baths and showers are unnecessary. Soothing creams will make the skin softer and will prevent much of the itching and skin irritation that occurs as a result of integumentary changes. Since alcohol further dries the skin, elderly persons should be instructed to read the labels on jars of creams and lotions carefully to make sure that the product does not contain this ingredient. Also a mild, nondrying soap should be used. Bath oils may be a good treatment for dry skin, but remember that they are very hazardous when placed in tub bath water. Climbing out of an oily bath tub is an excellent way to acquire a nasty fracture. Oil may, however, be applied to the moist skin following the tub bath, which also provides quicker absorption. When a bed bath is being given, oil may be added to the bath water.

Everyone worries about the appearance of his or her hair and face. In these areas the effects of aging are most evident. Men are most often burdened by the loss of scalp hair, although this also happens to women. There are many causes of baldness, including racial tendencies, genetic factors, and hormonal changes. Balding may begin with greying, progressing to total loss of hair color, followed by gradual but steady thinning out of the hair. Balding may begin at any age; it is not exclusively a problem of the elderly. There are only two solutions: One is to live with it; the other is to cover it. Wigs and hairpieces are available in a wide range of prices and styles. They are considered most fashionable, and if they make the elderly more comfortable about their appearance, the investment is worthwhile.

Many women over sixty notice that they are sprouting chin hairs, which is particularly offensive to them, since facial hair is considered most unfeminine. Scissors, tweezers, a razor, or a facial depilatory will quickly solve this problem. Again, a word of caution: Remember that unsteady hands, poor vision, and a sharp instrument combine to create a potentially dangerous situation. Facial depilatories can be very irritating to delicate skin tissue, and these should be used with extreme care.

When you look at the face of an aging person, you very readily observe many wrinkles and crow's-feet. These features begin to develop early in life—in the twenties—and are caused by the constant use of the same facial expressions over a lengthy period of time. Prolonged exposure to the sun will hasten the development of these characteristics, especially in very fair-skinned people. Loss of fat and elastic fiber can be observed in the face. The skin droops, a double chin develops, and the lower lids become puffy. The skin also has a grayish appearance, which may be caused by decreased capillaries and a lack of fresh air and exercise.

Careful and skillful use of cosmetics can disguise many of the signs of aging. However, creams, lotions, and ointments that promise a rebirth of youthful skin can only create false hope. Some men and women have plastic surgery performed for cosmetic purposes. Very often national magazines publish articles written by movie or television celebrities reporting the wonderful results obtained from facial uplift surgery. This procedure is very expensive and is not generally available to the ordinary person.

By the time one reaches the age of sixty-five his or her facial features reveal a great deal about his years of living. Crow's-feet, for example, are nothing more than happiness lines. When an elderly person laughs, these wrinkles are truly a part of his facial characteristics, a part of the person he "really" is.

The integumentary system gives proof that the growth process still continues during aging. This can be noted in the growth of fingernails and toenails. The toenails may become hardened and very thick, almost impossible to cut. Soaking the feet in warm water and applying cocoa butter or lanolin to the skin, cuticles, and nails helps to soften them, but the aged are advised to have thick, horny toenails cut by a podiatrist. Any injury to the tissues of the toes and feet can cause major problems for the elderly. Poor circulation in the lower limbs leaves the older person particularly vulnerable to slow healing, ulceration, infection, and gangrene in this area. The nurse is advised not to tackle the problem of toenail cutting, but to institute a referral to the podiatrist or foot clinic.

In summary, the aging process affects the integumentary system most visibly. These changes, however, do not present severe physical problems; rather they present problems of self-image. We are living in a era when aging is most unacceptable and signs of growing old are continually camouflaged. The aged person who is valued for who and what he is, rather than for what he looks like, will adjust to his appearance readily and be satisfied with his self-image.

NERVOUS SYSTEM CHANGES

One phenomenon that occurs during the process of aging is common to all body systems: a decrease in functioning cellular activity. The number of basic functioning units in the nervous system is reduced.

Many people tend to think that the aging process is confined to a few years in the sixties and seventies. However, a steady loss of neurons that characterizes aging in the nervous system begins surprisingly early, probably at the age of twenty-five.[4] This reduction of cell function accelerates as one grows older. Nerve fibers begin to degenerate as increased amounts of connective tissue appear.

Because of the smaller number of neurons, resulting in reduced nerve bundles and fibers, the capacity for transmitting impulses to and from the brain is also reduced. The speed with which the body reacts to stimuli, or the person's reaction time, is slowed. A contributing factor is the older adult's decreased physical activity, which results in decreased muscle tone.

Slower reaction time has implications for the older automobile driver, and he should realistically assess his ability to respond to sudden dangers on the road. Realizing one's limitations and acting accordingly may prevent serious accidents. The elderly should be cautioned against driving when road conditions are hazardous; even the best driver has difficulty driving in rain, snow, or fog. Driving at dusk or at night should be avoided, since the eyes of older people have difficulty in adjusting to shadows and dim lights. Even when the road conditions are good, taking the car out during peak rush hours puts a tax on the nervous system of young and old alike. For the older person, with his reduced reaction time, this can be dangerous. In order to compensate for his slower response, the older driver is usually much more cautious than others. He has a tendency to drive so slowly that the impatient motorist behind him may become exasperated and take suicidal chances in order to pass. However, there is no reason for the elderly person to discontinue driving provided routine physical exams by the physician indicate that he has the ability to handle it.

Some people may question whether the loss of functioning neurons affects a person's intellectual capabilities. Research has shown no impairment, but rather has shown stable intelligence levels over a period of many years. A look through the local newspaper, usually in June, will reveal articles on the seventy-five-year-old grandmother graduating from college with her twenty-one-year-old grandson. Although this case may be the exceptional one, it does show that the older person retains his intellectual capabilities. Under stressful situations, however, he may find it more difficult to reason out a problem. Coping with stress is a problem for everyone no matter what age, but the older person appears to be less able to handle it.

The lay public seems to automatically equate advancing age with senility, as if it were an inevitable consequence. This is a misconception that the nurse can help to eliminate. The fear that older persons have of losing their intellectual capacity needs to be allayed. Although the blood supply to the brain decreases significantly in the elderly, there is no correlation between decreased blood flow to the brain and senility. Senility, then, is not an inevitable process of aging. This disease process will be discussed fully in Chapter 9.

As we know, nerves and nerve fibers serve to relay impulses to and from the brain. In the elderly the ability of these nerves to transport messages is decreased. Sensory nerve endings in the skin may be less alert to stimuli, as illustrated by the diminished ability to react to the hot-water bottle that is too hot. The motor nerves that simulate muscles to contract in order to move part of the body are also affected. Muscle tone, the state of readiness of the muscle to contract fully, is decreased as well. The elderly person should be aware of the decrease in sensory and motor conduction and situations that obviously call for quick responses.

Physical inactivity not only contributes to decreased muscle tone, but can also lead to insomnia, a common coping problem of the aged. Although insomnia is not peculiar to the aged, many times it becomes more pronounced. A common misconception is that the aged need increased amounts of sleep. Although they need increased periods of rest, sleep requirements for the healthy older person do not change. Sleep interrupted by waking several times during the night can be most disturbing. Contributing factors may be physical inactivity, anxiety, long naps during the day, boredom, or excessive mental stimulation before retiring. The elderly should be cautioned against the use of nonprescribed, commercially prepared drugs that induce sleep. Some of these drugs are not eliminated from the body fast enough and cause morning drowsiness and a hangover effect, which can be very dangerous. If sedatives are needed, the physician is the only one qualified to determine the specific medication and dosage required. The older person can be assisted in evaluating his daily plan of activities to assure adequate time for rest. Perhaps he can set aside an hour in the afternoon for a nap.

As the aging process continues, the sense organs that appear to be the most vulnerable to change are the eye and ear. Damage to the transparent portions of the eye results in reduced visual ability. The ciliary muscles become more rigid, and with this comes a loss in the eye's power of accommodation. The ability of the eye to react quickly to darkness is reduced, and the difficulty in adjusting to dim light is even greater.

Loss of peripheral vision as well as the ability to discriminate color has real implications for coping with everyday situations. Elderly pedestrians need to be cautioned not to rely on side vision but to turn their head and look both ways before crossing the street. Objects should be placed directly in front of the person rather than off to the side. Because of the older person's difficulty in distinguishing similar colors, accidents in the home can be reduced by carpeting and wall colors of contrasting shades. Reds and yellows, for example, are easier to see than blues and greens. If doors are painted a color that contrasts with the surrounding walls, they will be more easily visible. Hazardous areas in the home can be made less dangerous by using proper color to alert the elderly. Many accidents in public buildings could also be avoided if interior decorators used this knowledge in their planning.

Since the aged person has difficulty seeing the water level in a clear water glass, it should only be half filled to prevent spilling. Also, the elderly person who has problems with his vision may not see a white tablet of medication placed on a white tablecloth. The tablet should be placed in the palm of the person's hand or in containers that can be readily seen.

The majority of elderly people require glasses for close work. Although many admit they cannot see well, they shy away from seeking medical attention because of the cost. They shop for glasses in the local store as they would for shoes. If the glasses fit all right, they take them. Buying eyeglasses in this way can be very harmful to the eye. Furthermore, accidents resulting from poor vision are numerous, since the elderly tend to rely more heavily on visual stimulation than a younger person. The difficulty in eye accommodation accompanied by diminished sensory-motor coordination can make stair climbing a hazard, and stairs should be provided with hand rails on both sides.

Routine eye examinations by the physician should include tests for the presence of glaucoma and for retinal changes, since arteriosclerosis of the retina is usually present. Many senior citizens' organizations offer free eye examinations routinely.

The physical appearance of the eye may be disturbing to the elderly person also. Although there are atrophic changes in the fibrous and elastic tissues of the eyelid, resulting in relaxation of the lower lid particularly, these changes do not result in impaired vision. The person may notice the presence of a grayish white ring around the iris. This condition is called arcus senilis and does not indicate the presence of disease in the eye. It is simply an indication of the aging process. Fading of the pigment of the iris is also a sign of this process. Weakened muscles controlling the eyelid accompanied by reduced amounts of fatty tissues around the orbit of the eye result in cosmetic changes. These are irreversible and do not affect the normal functioning of the eye.

Impairment of hearing is a more common complaint among the elderly than the problems of visual acuity. Physiological changes include degeneration of auditory nerve fiber, thickening of the eardrum, and decreased production of cerumen. It is interesting to note that throughout life there continues to be a progressive decrease in our hearing ability. Although these changes are slight, they do exist.

The ability to hear tones within the range of normal conversational levels is diminished, and the aging ear has more difficulty in picking up normal speech sounds. The central nervous system, in turn, has difficulty in interpreting the information relayed by the ear. It has been estimated that one out of every four persons over sixty has a hearing loss sufficient for one to use the term "deaf." Otosclerosis and cochlear fibrosis are contributing factors.

Yearly physical examination should include audiometric studies. For some causes of deafness, the use of a hearing aid may be helpful. If the elderly person does not want to try the hearing aid, however, forcing the issue is of no use. The aid may be properly fitted and properly functioning but of no value if it sits in the bureau drawer along with the dentures and eyeglasses.

Just as eyeglasses need adjustments, so do hearing aids, and they should be checked at intervals to assure correct functioning. With the advances made in electronic technology, hearing aids come in a variety of models and can be worn almost invisibly.

The nurse can assist the family of the hard-of-hearing person by giving them the following helpful pointers in dealing with problems of communication. Stand directly facing the person. Lower your voice and use clear distinct speech. Do not use exaggerated speech or mouth the words. Introduce the subject for discussion with a single preliminary remark. Speak on a subject that is familiar to the individual. Hard-of-hearing persons who lip-read find it easier if your face is not in the shadows but clearly visible. If these simple rules are followed, the hard of hearing will understand the conversation more readily. Shouting confuses the elderly and creates the impression of disapproval. It is a needless frustrating experience for both listener and speaker.

The nurse may suggest to the hard-of-hearing person that he enroll in a class to learn to lip-read. Evening adult schools and speech and hearing clinics offer these services.

STUDY QUESTIONS AND PROBLEMS

1. Take a quick but observant tour of your home and note anything that could be hazardous to the elderly. Prepare a list of these hazards and ways in which they could be corrected. Discuss in class.

2. Mrs. Casey has given her husband the following list of jobs to be done around the house: remove storm windows and put up screens; paint the back porch; and clean the cellar. These are all strenuous activities. How can they be spaced to avoid exertion?

3. Mr. Gedney is an avid television fan. He has not missed a televised sports event in his ten years of retirement. His TV day starts with the first afternoon ball game and ends with the late, late show. He sits in a cloud of cigarette smoke, leaving the television set only to go to the bathroom. He eats his dinner on a tray as the action continues. Discuss the effects of Mr. Gedney's daily routine on the circulatory-respiratory and skeletomuscular systems.

4. Mr. and Mrs. Roberts sleep until 10:00 A.M. each day. They eat a brunch of sweet rolls and coffee at 11:00 A.M. and a dinner of meat, mashed potatoes, gravy, and cake or pie for dessert. Their evening is spent watching TV and munching on crackers and drinking cola or beer. Evaluate Mr. and Mrs. Roberts' diet.

5. Mr. and Mrs. Harrington have planned a trip to visit their children. The five-hundred-mile trip by turnpike is of concern to the couple, since they both experience urinary frequency and urgency. What can they do to solve this problem?

6. Since the elderly person reacts less quickly in emergencies, what precautionary measures might be taken to assure his readiness to deal with the following situations?
   a. grease fire in the oven
   b. electrical blackout
   c. flat tire on the freeway

7. What facilities that are available in your community provide the following services for the aged:
   a. foot care
   b. vision testing
   c. diabetic screening
   d. nutrition counseling
   e. free chest X ray

BIBLIOGRAPHY

Anderson, Helen C. *Newton's Geriatric Nursing.* 5th ed. Saint Louis: C. V. Mosby, 1971.

Birren, James E., ed. *Handbook of Aging and The Individual.* Chicago: University of Chicago Press, 1959.

Blumenthal, Herman T., ed. *Medical and Clinical Aspects of Aging.* New York: Columbia University Press, 1962.

Buckley, Joseph C. *The Retirement Handbook.* 3rd ed. New York: Harper & Row, 1967.

Burgess, Ernest W., ed. *Aging in Western Societies.* Chicago: University of Chicago Press, 1960.

Gilbert, Jeanne. *Understanding Old Age.* New York: Ronald Press, 1952.

Howell, Trevor H. *A Student's Guide to Geriatrics.* Springfield, Ill.: Charles C. Thomas, 1963.

Masters, William H., and Johnson, Virginia E. *Human Sexual Response*. Boston: Little, Brown, 1966.

Mitchell, H. S.; Rynbergen, H. J.; Anderson, L.; and Dibble, M. V. *Cooper's Nutrition in Health and Disease*. 25th ed. Philadelphia: J. B. Lippincott, 1968.

Palmore, Erdman, ed. *Normal Aging. Reports from the Duke Longitudinal Study, 1955–1969*. Durham, N. C.: Duke University Press, 1970.

Peyton, Alice. *Practical Nutrition*. 2nd ed. Philadelphia: J. B. Lippincott, 1962.

Prehoda, Robert W. *Extended Youth*. New York: G. P. Putnam's Sons, 1968.

Rossman, Isadore, ed. *Clinical Geriatrics*. Philadelphia: J. B. Lippincott, 1971.

Rothenberg, Robert E. *Health in the Later Years*. New York: New American Library, 1964.

Rubin, Isadore. *Sexual Life After Sixty*. New York: Basic Books, 1965.

Shafer, Kathleen N.; Sawyer, Janet R.; McCluskey, Audrey M.; Beck, Edna L.; Phipps, Wilma J. *Medical-Surgical Nursing*. 5th ed. Saint Louis: C. V. Mosby, 1971.

Smith, Dorothy; Germain, Carol; and Gips, Claudia. *Care of the Adult Patient*. 3rd ed. Philadelphia: J. B. Lippincott, 1971.

U.S., Department of Health, Education, and Welfare, *Working with Older People—A Guide to Practice*, vol. 1, *The Practitioner and the Elderly*. Washington, D.C.: U.S. Government Printing Office, 1970.

U.S., Department of Health, Education, and Welfare, *Working with Older People—A Guide to Practice*, vol. 2, *Biological, Psychological and Sociological Aspects of Aging*. Washington, D.C.: U.S. Government Printing Office, 1970.

U.S., Department of Health, Education, and Welfare, *Working with Older People—A Guide to Practice*, vol 3. *The Aging Person: Needs and Services*. Washington, D.C.: U.S. Government Printing Office, 1970.

NOTES

1. Vera J. and Jerome S. Peterson, *Aging in Western Societies*, ed. Ernest W. Burgess (Chicago: University of Chicago Press, 1960), p. 156.
2. Isadore Rossman, ed. *Clinical Geriatrics* (Philadelphia: J. B. Lippincott, 1971), p. 3.
3. William H. Masters and Virginia E. Johnson, *Human Sexual Response* (Boston: Little, Brown, 1966), p. 270.
4. Alan Barham Carter, "The Neurologic Aspects of Aging," in *Clinical Geriatrics*, ed. Isadore Rossman (Philadelphia: J. B. Lippincott, 1971), p. 123.

5

Illness in the Later Years

The incidence of illness is highest among older adults due to degenerative changes occurring in all body systems. Illness can be classified in terms of duration of time and severity—short- or long-term, major or minor. Short-term illness can be defined as an illness requiring care for less than thirty days in a general hospital or at home. It may be of an acute nature and lead eventually to complications resulting in a long-term illness. Examples of short-term illnesses include upper respiratory infections and appendicitis. Long-term illness requires a prolonged period of care—at least thirty days in a general hospital or more time in an institution or home. An example of an illness requiring long-term care is a cerebral vascular accident. Some illnesses of long-term duration may also be classified as chronic. In addition to requiring long-term care, a chronic illness results in one or more of the following: permanent impairment, residual disability, irreversible pathological alterations, and the necessity for special rehabilitative training.

Whatever the degree of severity, illness takes its toll physically and emotionally on the aged. Illness, particularly long-term, is especially dreaded by older persons, who are vulnerable both psychologically and financially. They react to symptoms of illness in the same way that they have dealt with such symptoms in the past. Some respond immediately by seeking medical help. Others make endless excuses for not seeing the doctor. High on the list of excuses are:

    1. "The doctor is too expensive. I just can't afford it."

2."Oh, it's a part of growing old—must be my rheumatism."
Health care insurance has contributed greatly to easing the financial burden, but still the elderly, as well as the young, find that illness can result in a real drain on the pocketbook. Long-term illness can eat up the elderly's lifetime savings, causing the one thing that many elderly people dread—financial dependence upon relatives.

Thus, signs of illness are disregarded, while the disease process continues unchecked. Home remedies and proprietary medicines, which are easily obtained at the local drugstore, are used by older adults in the hope that symptoms will disappear. Television commercials have played a big part in fostering the concept of immediate results. Only when symptoms become extremely severe do some elderly persons relent and seek the help they need.

Lack of transportation may be another reason for their delaying the trip to the doctor's office or clinic. Many elderly persons have difficulty using public transportation even if it is readily available to them. Communities are now developing services to provide the elderly with transportation to a doctor's office. By calling a central phone number, the patient can have a vehicle pick him up at his home, deliver him to the clinic or doctor's office, and return him to his home after the appointment.

Another factor contributing to the person's delay in getting professional help may be fear of what the doctor will find. "Perhaps it's cancer." "I'll be a cripple the rest of my life." "Maybe I'm going to die." These thoughts keep running through the older person's mind.

Although any illness can be disrupting to the patient and his family, short-term illnesses can be more easily tolerated. It is the prolonged illness that has serious effects on the patient, his family, and the ones administering care. Restorative nursing and specific long-term illnesses will be discussed in succeeding chapters.

THE PATIENT'S CHOICE OF A PLACE OF CARE

The long-term patient, then, is one that has a chronic disease or impairments that require care over a prolonged period of time. Since the physician's supervision and assistance from members of the health care team are necessary before the patient can learn to assume a greater responsibility for self-care and independence, the physician may want him to be admitted to a general hospital, where continuous care can be given. Continuous care may also be obtained in an extended care facility, nursing home, or the patient's own home.

It is estimated that there are approximately 1.7 million geriatric patients requiring long-term care. Once the physician has diagnosed the condition as one requiring care over a prolonged period of time, the immediate question becomes, "Where can this care be given?" There are many factors that influence the answer to this question, the nature of the illness being a major one. As a result of some illnesses, the patient may become completely dependent on others for his physical care; in other situations, however, he may be able to assume responsibility for self-care with some assistance. Thus, the following questions arise: Must the patient be confined to bed, or is he able to ambulate? How dependent is he on others? Does the nature of the illness warrant admission to a general hospital or to a rehabilitation center where the patient can join an active rehabilitation program? The physician's judgment and recommendations should be a major factor in answering these questions.

Although the physician may recommend the location—be it general hospital, rehabilitation center, nursing home, or the patient's home— the patient's and his family's attitudes toward the recommended site can be another influencing factor. The mere thought of having to leave the comfort and security of his home and loved ones may pose a real threat to the patient. "Leave me alone. I'd rather die at home than in some strange place," may be his attitude. Another, wishing not to burden his family, will readily accept the decision for him to be admitted to a health care facility. However, although the patient may have a positive attitude toward going to a long-term health care facility, he is also influenced by the attitudes of his family and friends. The family may feel that placing the patient in a home, no matter how excellent, would be a disgrace—that it would indicate the patient was no longer loved. Care at the patient's own home would then seem to be the only answer. Although the home environment provides the patient with an atmosphere that is not foreign to him and hopefully with a setting where he is surrounded by those who love him, the real question remains: Can the program of rehabilitation be carried out effectively? Can the continuity of care that is required be provided at home without completely disrupting the family unit? The patient and his family will require assistance in answering these questions honestly and objectively.

Selection of the health care facility is also dependent on the patient's and/or his family's financial ability. Medicare or nongovernmental insurance policies may help pay for the major part of the costs. Insurance policies do have restrictions, however, and the wording of the policy may be confusing. The insurance agent should explain what costs are covered and what costs are not in language that is easily understood by the patient, spouse, and other family members. Those eligible under Medicare can contact the local Social Security office about specific questions, and the local welfare office will provide details regarding Medicaid eligibility. It has been said that the extent of the patient's insurance coverage determines where he will receive care more often than his medical condition and needs. This is unfortunate in many cases but true.

Determining what resources are available for providing long-term care can be a frustrating experience for all concerned. If the patient and family decide on home care, there may be community agencies whose role is to assist in the patient's care and rehabilitation. The physician may order home visits by a physical therapist, a speech therapist, or the nursing personnel of a public health nursing agency or a visiting nurse association. Sometimes home care programs are sponsored by the local hospital or health department and coordinate the services that the patient requires. If the disabled person lives alone or had been the family's homemaker, the services of the local homemaker agency may also be required.

If care outside the patient's home is indicated, the patient and family will need to determine the availability of health care facilities in the area. The family physician should be consulted for his recommendations. The health care worker should also be knowledgeable about community resources and about county and state facilities. Local social service agencies and public health departments have listings of agencies, including addresses, type of licensure or accreditation, and other information helpful to the patient and his family. The patient and his family will need to know whether the institution under consideration meets the criteria for approval under Medicare legislation.

In selecting the appropriate facility, the patient and family should visit the institution if possible. The American Nursing Home Association has pamphlets that outline what one should look for in a tour of a nursing home and what questions one should ask of the administration.

The type of sponsorship of the institution, whether voluntary, public, or proprietary, should also be known. The family should avoid nonlicensed institutions, since these do not meet even the minimum standards for safety and care established in the state and are not approved institutions for Medicare beneficiaries and/or Medicaid patients.

Cost factors need to be carefully weighed. The cheapest facility may not, in reality, be so cheap, due to hidden costs that are not discussed during the initial visit. The basic daily rate may be low, but the "extras" can add up.

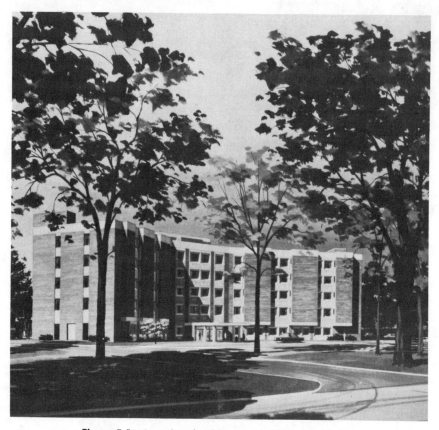

Figure 5-1: A modern health and rehabilitation facility.

Once the health care facility has been selected and the patient admitted, the problem of who will give the care has been solved. However, the patient and his family will have to make new adjustments to the illness, its effects, and the institution.

THE PATIENT'S NEED FOR INDIVIDUALIZED CARE

Throughout this text the need to maintain a meaningful life has been stressed. Illness in any degree of severity can have a drastic effect on this developmental task. Any illness will cause a certain amount of dependency, and this dependency occurs at a time when the individual's need to be independent is more intense than at any other period except adolescence.[1] He may be dependent on his spouse, the general hospital, the extended care facility, and/or a host of health care workers. The patient is removed from his normal activities, on a temporary or permanent basis, and is unable to maintain his sense of usefulness by contributing to the community.

The elderly view illness as a catastrophe, and so it can be—physically, emotionally, socially, and economically. Fear is a companion that accompanies any disease condition. Fear of dying is the foremost fear of the aged. Moreover, they are afraid of dying alone and abandoned by their loved ones. Any health care institution represents the place where this may happen ("Oh, the nursing home—that's where they put you to die.")

The aged, like everybody else, are afraid of the unknown. The fear is more 'pronounced among these patients because they adjust slowly to new surroundings and situations. This slowness in adjusting is often manifested by confused or disoriented behavior, which many health workers attribute to senility. Usually this is a false assumption. Given a little time and clear, truthful explanations, the patient will adjust very well to his surroundings. However, institutional routines can contribute to confusion and anxiety. The admitting office, for example, demands that the patient recall past illnesses and remember specific information concerning relatives—mother, father, spouse—who may have been deceased for years. Painful memories of loved ones are brought back into focus at a time when the institution is asking the patient to sign legal forms having important significance for his future. No wonder this overwhelming experience can aggravate feelings of insecurity and anxiety. Certainly, institutions should revise their admitting office procedures and obtain only the most essential information in an atmosphere and manner that are less confusing and emotionally taxing on the patient.

When the patient is transported to the nursing unit, he must go through other routines that begin to strip away his individuality. Think of the modest elderly patient who has to replace his street clothes with the white, short hospital gown, open in the back with only ties to hold both sides together. How embarrassed and humiliated he must feel. Is the nursing staff flexible enough to permit the patient to wear his own bedclothes or his own underclothes under the hospital gown? Or must all patients conform to the set standards? Is the staff willing to allow the patient to wear his favorite cap—day and night—or to carry his well-used pipe? Is the staff considerate of the patient's life-style, so that he retains a part of his own identity as an individual human being? Many times the nurse becomes so concerned with procedures and routines that human, individualized care is somehow forgotten. For example, she may be so absorbed in placing side rails on the bed that she fails to explain to the patient why they are needed. Without an explanation, the patient may feel that he is being closed up or locked out of a world with which he is familiar. What a threat to a man's dignity!

Before the patient is oriented to his surroundings, he may have difficulty understanding the institution's call-light system. Pushing a button at his bedside to alert a nurse down the hall may be most confusing to him, and as a result, he may not use the call light when he needs assistance. The nursing staff should be able to devise an alternative method for meeting his needs.

Initially patients are addressed by their surname and title, but as the nurse and patient build up mutual respect and understanding, the patient should be asked what he would like to be called and what he would like to call the nurse. Perhaps it has been many years since the patient has been called by his first name. Those who would have used his first name may no longer be around, and the patient's family would use titles like Dad and Grandfather. He may prefer to hear his own name once again. Whatever title is used, it is agreed upon by both patient and nurse as a personal relationship is built. This does not mean that all the staff members will call the patient by the same title, since the relationship between the patient and each staff member will not be the same.

When the elderly person is hospitalized, his opportunities to make choices are severely limited. Whenever possible, he should be given the opportunity to make choices about such things as eating in the dining room or in his own room, participating in group recreation or not. In many instances the patient is given no choice in these matters and is pushed from one activity to the next as if he were a thing rather than an individual human being.

If we are to humanize geriatric care, we need to consider the life-style of each individual patient and pattern our care plan with this vital information in mind. Only then will the care we give make a real difference to the patient and, therefore, to ourselves.

The patient's adjustment to the physical environment of the institution will be quicker if the care plan takes into consideration his mode of living prior to his hospitalization. However, the patient's adjustment to his illness and its consequences and resulting limitations, if there are any, is not quite as easy. It is not difficult to accept the fact that one has a common cold and to live with the limitations caused by it. But adjusting to a cerebral vascular accident and accepting the consequences (such as hemiplegia or aphasia) and the limitations caused by it is another matter.

Patients react to devastating and long-term illnesses in many ways. It is not uncommon for the patient to experience anger, which is often expressed in open hostility toward health care workers. The entire patient care team should discuss this hostile behavior and their reactions to it, and plan an approach that will allow the patient to feel accepted. Hostility may also arise because the older adult views the health care worker as a representative of the younger generation (a constant reminder of lost youth), as a torturer who moves and turns him even though it hurts, or as a domineering, bossy person who constantly nags and picks on him, giving him no peace. What a shock to learn that all patients do not view those who care for them as angels of mercy with soothing hands and voices.

Most people live up to what others expect of them. If the health care worker expects the aged patient to be confused or to act in a childish manner, the patient probably will act accordingly. If the aged are approached with the attitude that they are responsible, esteemed, intelligent, capable of understanding, and entitled to explanations of what is happening, they tend to behave accordingly.[2]

The aged frequently experience loneliness and social isolation. Many of these people have a life-span that has extended beyond that of their friends and loved ones. Extended care facilities seem to have replaced extended families. But little has been done to help the older person have meaningful social relationships in these institutions.[3] Those who work in such facilities would agree with the wisdom of getting the patient out of bed every day. However, it is one thing to get out of bed and another to have something to do when one gets out of bed! The time out of bed could be a time for social activity and interaction instead of television watching or just sitting. Wheelchairs should not be lined up along the wall. Remember that the aged person has decreased peripheral vision and may not see the person next to him. Wheelchairs should be opposite one another to stimulate conversation and socializing. Residents of long-term care facilities should find companionship and friendship among fellow patients and the staff.

Open and unrestricted visiting hours in nursing homes and extended care facilities provide the opportunity for the patient and his family to maintain close contact. The aged person who is lonely and feels that his family "put me here to get rid of me" may vent his anger on the family. To spare themselves emotional scenes, the family may stop visiting the patient entirely. This action will only compound the problem by reinforcing the patient's beliefs and increasing his anger and loneliness. The health care worker should discuss this situation with the nursing team leader. Efforts should be made to help the family understand the reasons for the patient's behavior, and frequent visits should be encouraged.

Some families feel guilty because they have placed a loved one in a long-term care facility. These guilt feelings may be manifested by resentment directed at the staff. "The care is not good enough." "The sheets are wrinkled"—nothing the staff can do or say is good enough. This is a difficult situation to tolerate, but the health care worker must try to understand the reasons for the family's behavior. Usually, it is not the patient who is complaining, and he may be genuinely embarrassed by the actions of his loved ones. The health care personnel must never react by taking it out on the patient. It is not his fault, and he needs some reassurance that the staff members understand that his family is concerned and wants to see that he has the best of care.

There are some families that are glad to be rid of the burden of the elderly sick. These people will not bother the staff or the patient; their sole contribution will be financial. To be forgotten by one's sons and daughters is heartbreaking, and the staff must provide the love that the aged person needs. In the article "It's Tough to Be Old," one elderly person confides: "Now I need security and understanding and hope. I need respect too, but most of all I need love."[4]

The health care worker in a geriatric facility assumes many roles: He is a supporter, a guide and companion through the unknown, and most important, a fellow human being. He or she must communicate clearly, give honest reassurances, and not be afraid to put his arm around the patient to physically comfort him. All those working with the aged sick should have as their goal the physical, social, and psychological well-being of the patient, and should help the patient to take pleasure from everyday life in a meaningful positive way.

STUDY QUESTIONS AND PROBLEMS

1. Prepare a list of licensed nursing homes in your area. Which ones are approved for Medicare recipients?
2. With your classmates, prepare a checklist of things to look for in the selection of a nursing home. Arrange a visit to one of the nursing homes in your area. Use the checklist to evaluate the facility.
3. Review any health insurance policies held by you or your family. Discuss their provisions in class.
4. Plan some activities that would increase social relationships among ambulatory patients confined to a nursing home.

BIBLIOGRAPHY

Anderson, Helen C. *Newton's Geriatric Nursing.* 5th ed. Saint Louis: C. V. Mosby, 1971.
Beland, Irene. *Clinical Nursing: Pathophysiological and Psychosocial Approaches.* 2nd ed. New York: Macmillan, 1970.

Burnside, Irene M. "Clocks and Calendars." *American Journal of Nursing,* January 1970.

Commission on Chronic Illness. *Chronic Illness in the United States,* vol. 2: *Care of the Long Term Patient.* Cambridge, Mass.: Harvard University Press, 1956.

Davis, Robert. "Psychologic Aspects of Geriatric Nursing." *American Journal of Nursing,* April 1968.

Falck, Hans, and Kane, Mary. *It Can't Be Home—Social and Emotional Aspects of Residential Care.* National Institute of Mental Health. Washington, D.C.: U.S. Government Printing Office, 1971.

Frenay, Sister Agnes Clare, and Pierce, Gloria. "The Climate of Care for a Geriatric Patient." *American Journal of Nursing,* September 1971, pp. 1747–1750.

Hahn, Aloyse. "It's Tough to Be Old." *American Journal of Nursing,* August 1970, pp. 1698–1699.

Hays, Joyce Sanhammer, and Larson, Kenneth. *Interacting with Patients.* New York: Macmillan, 1964.

Hirschberg, Gerald G.; Lewis, Leon; and Thomas, Dorothy. *Rehabilitation: A Manual for the Care of the Disabled and Elderly.* Philadelphia: J. B. Lippincott, 1964.

Hofling, Charles K., and Leninger, Madeline M. *Basic Psychiatric Concepts in Nursing.* Philadelphia: J. B. Lippincott, 1967.

Hudson, Joan Howard. "Decision." *American Journal of Nursing,* April 1970.

Moody, Linda; Baron, Virginia; and Monk, Grace. "Moving the Past into the Present." *American Journal of Nursing,* November 1970.

Roth, Julius, and Eddy, Elizabeth. *Rehabilitation for the Unwanted.* New York: Atherton Press, 1967.

Schoenberg, Bernard; Carr, Arthur C.; Peretz, David; and Kutscher, Austin H. (editors). *Loss and Grief: Psychological Management in Medical Practice.* New York: Columbia University Press, 1970.

Smith, Dorothy; Germain, Carol H.; and Gips, Claudia. *Care of the Adult Patient.* 3rd ed. Philadelphia: J. B. Lippincott, 1971.

Stone, Virginia. "Give the Older Person Time." *American Journal of Nursing,* October 1969.

Terry, Florence Jones, et al. *Principles and Techniques of Rehabilitation.* Saint Louis: C. V. Mosby, 1957.

Thinking About a Nursing Home. Washington, D.C.: American Nursing Home Association, 1971.

NOTES

1. Robert Davis, "Psychologic Aspects of Geriatric Nursing," *American Journal of Nursing,* April 1968, p. 803.
2. Ibid.
3. Linda Moody, Virginia Baron, and Grace Monk, "Moving the Past into the Present," *American Journal of Nursing,* November 1970, p. 2353.
4. Aloyse Hahn, "It's Tough to Be Old," *American Journal of Nursing,* August 1970, p. 1699.

6

Restorative Nursing

Restorative nursing is an integral part of nursing care for all patients. It is not unique to the care of the aged. The goal of restorative nursing activities is to return the patient to the community as a contributing, functioning member of society. Many believe that restorative care begins when the patient is admitted to a special rehabilitation center. Actually, this phase of nursing begins with the diagnosis of disease and continues until the patient gains as much physical independence as possible.

Since World War II there has been an increased awareness of the need for rehabilitative processes. During this period the health care community has come to realize that promptness of restorative care is a vital factor in the improvement or attainment of lost physical functions. Today, in some geographic areas the demand for restorative therapy is exceeding the ability of professionals to deliver such services. In many instances several institutions share the services of a physical therapist, occupational therapist, and speech therapist. This demand has given rise to new categories of health care workers, such as occupational therapy assistants, physical therapy assistants, and others who are prepared in one- to two-year programs and function as assistants to rehabilitation professionals. Restorative nursing activities—whether they are an independent function of one nursing team member or part of a coordinated effort—are a major component of any program of therapy.

Physically disabled persons have some difficulty with the functioning of their muscular, skeletal, and nervous systems. This malfunctioning can be classified into one of the following groups:

1. Temporary disability, in which the lost function is expected to return, and the disability can be corrected. The period of convalescence may be short or long. Examples would be a fractured hip or dislocated shoulder.
2. Permanent disability, in which the lost function cannot be restored but can be replaced with substitutions. Examples of substitutions would be an artificial limb following amputation or eyeglasses that replace an opaque crystalline lens (cataract) following surgery.
3. Progressive disability, in which the function diminishes over a period of time and will never return. It cannot be replaced, and no substitutions can be made. Examples of this would be multiple sclerosis, muscular dystrophy, and rheumatoid arthritis.

The basic foundation of the rehabilitation program is quality nursing care, which the patient receives from the onset of the illness. This informal phase of rehabilitation is aimed at preventing complications that would retard the patient's progress toward rehabilitation. Proper bed positioning to prevent contractures, frequent turning of the patient to prevent decubitus ulcers, and meticulous skin care are a few of the many nursing measures that are important aspects of the beginning rehabilitation regimen.

THE ACTIVE REHABILITATION PROGRAM

The formal rehabilitation process begins with the evaluation of the patient and his need for therapy. The decision to undertake a program of active rehabilitation is a serious one because of the risks involved. In some cases the risks in undergoing this process may far outweigh the possible benefits. These risks include further damage to an already injured part, undue stress and strain on other body systems, injury resulting from falls, and the possibility of failure. For example, a patient with a fractured hip may benefit from learning how to use crutches, but the increased stress placed upon an already overburdened circulatory system may well produce more serious problems. In some cases the disease process may have progressed to the point where the return of function cannot be considered as a possibility or where the function cannot be replaced. The patient's age, general physical and emotional health, stamina, and attitudes toward rehabilitation are determining factors in the decision to institute a program of therapy. The most important person in the rehabilitative process is the patient himself. Because of the active role he must play in his recovery, it is essential for him to be interested, enthusiastic, and willing to attempt active participation. If he does not have these attitudes, all the efforts of the rehabilitation team will be useless.

It is unrealistic to assume that all patients are candidates for active rehabilitation. For those patients who will not benefit from therapy, care will be directed toward the goal of maintaining the existing function. It is important to realize that such custodial care is no less exacting than the care given to the acutely ill, and the principles of patient care discussed in this chapter should also be utilized when caring for the long-term patient who is not in active rehabilitation. The patient and his family need to know why it has been decided to forgo a progressive rehabilitation regimen and what plans for care will be made.

When the rehabilitation team decides a patient will benefit from an active rehabilitation process, the physician, who is always the team leader, plans the program of therapy along with other health professionals. Ideally, this physician will be a physiatrist—a doctor who has advanced preparation in the physical, mental, social, and economic aspects of rehabilitation. Other members of the team may be a physical therapist, occupational therapist, internist, recreational therapist, psychiatrist, social worker, speech and hearing therapist, rehabilitation nurse, public health nurse, and vocational rehabilitation counselor. Other personnel, such as a dietitian or pharmacist may be invited to attend the evaluation and planning conference if the patient's special needs warrant it. The entire rehabilitation team meets at regularly scheduled intervals to review the patient's progress and to adjust the therapy program as necessary.

When the patient begins to play an active role in his recovery, he shifts from total dependence and begins to gain increasing physical independence. The patient may be out of the nursing care unit for long periods of the day, returning only to nap or spend the evening and night. It is not unusual for the nursing staff to miss the close contact with the patient; sometimes nurses may even be jealous of the time that other rehabilitation team members spend with the patient. Patient care personnel must realize that the patient is not the property or sole responsibility of any one department. Rather, it is the responsibility of all rehabilitation personnel to function as a team that can win the patient's recovery.

Nursing personnel will find that their role will change as the patient's independence increases, although the nurse will continue to be the supportive and encouraging person in the nursing care unit. As the patient increases his skill and confidence, the nurse will reinforce the therapy by helping the patient to assume more self-care. Communication becomes increasingly more important, since pertinent information must be relayed to other members of the rehabilitation team. Also, the nurse must be able to answer the patient's questions regarding his therapy.

The nursing team will meet to develop methods for carrying out its special role in the rehabilitative program. These methods are called the nursing care plan. Team members include the head nurse and all others who share the responsibility for patient care.

Since the patient will spend most of his day away from the nursing unit, many activities that are traditionally the responsibility of the day shift will have to be assumed by the evening and night shifts. For example, the patient may bathe in the evening before retiring. Transportation to and from therapy departments will have to be planned. Will the patient be taken by wheelchair, wheel his own chair, or walk? If he walks will he be aided or go unassisted? As he progresses in therapy, will his mode of travel be changed? How can the nursing staff enhance and further extend the specific therapies being conducted? Of utmost importance is the determination of what is to be done for the patient and what the patient should do for himself.

The head nurse will report the patient's progress to the entire rehabilitation group when they meet for review and planning. The nursing care plan is a flexible approach to the patient's needs and is adjusted as he progresses.

THE PATIENT CONFINED TO BED

All those who are giving or assisting with nursing care should be aware that they are playing a vital role in the rehabilitation of the patient requiring long-term care. Dependency, deterioration, and depression are terms that are not compatible with the goals of the health care team. Rehabilitation may be a prolonged process, and in part it is dependent on measures taken immediately after the onset of the illness. For the patient confined to bed, one of the goals of nursing care must be the prevention of deformities. This can be accomplished by helping the patient to maintain the existing range of joint motion, seeing that he maintains proper body positioning, and frequently turning patients who need assistance in moving.

Maintaining the Patient's Range of Motion

The extent to which motion is possible at a particular joint depends on several factors: The type of joint (ball-and-socket or hinge), the disease processes affecting the area, the muscles surrounding the joint, and the ability of these muscles to extend and contract in order to produce movement. Range of motion, then, is the extent to which the joint is capable of being moved.

Loss of joint motion can also result from the person's hesitation to move painful joints. The position the patient assumes will be the one causing the least amount of discomfort. When the patient tends to use the same position over a period of time, one set of muscles and connective tissue surrounding the joint remains in a contracted state due to lack of use, and there is a permanent shortening of these muscle fibers. In this condition, known as a contracture, the joint is locked into one position, and the patient finds he can no longer move it into another. If the joint is locked into a bent position, the muscles causing the joint to straighten are not used, which creates a wasting away, or atrophy, of the muscle fibers. Prevention of contractures and muscle atrophy is a prime responsibility of the rehabilitation team. Range-of-motion exercises may be used to accomplish this goal and thus to prevent further barriers to the rehabilitative process. (See Figure 6-1.)

All who work at rehabilitation need a knowledge of the terms used to refer to the movements performed by healthy joints and muscles. The following basic movements are used in range-of-motion exercises:

1. Flexion: bending motion, or the moving of one body part toward the other. Hinge joints accomplish this movement. Example: bending the elbow so that the hand touches the shoulder.

2. Extension: stretching motion, or the moving of one body part away from the other in order to straighten out the body alignment. Hinge joints also accomplish this movement, which is the opposite of the flexion. Example: bringing the flexed elbow back to the straight position, or straightening the elbow.

3. Abduction: movement *away* from the center of the body or one of its parts. Example: moving the arms away from normal position at the side of the body.

4. Adduction: movement *toward* the center of the body or one of its parts. This movement is the opposite of abduction. Example: moving the arm from the normal position at the side of the body toward the center of the body.

5. Internal rotation: movement turning inward toward the center. This movement is accomplished by ball-and-socket joints. Example: rotating the leg inward so that the knee is facing the other leg.

6. External rotation: movement turning outward from the center. This movement is also accomplished by ball-and-socket joints and

is the opposite of internal rotation. Example: rotating the leg outward so that the knee is facing away from the other leg.

7. Pronation: movement turning downward. Example: With the forearm in horizontal position, rotating the forearm so that the palm of the hand is facing downward.

8. Supination: movement turning upward. Example: With the forearm in horizontal position, rotating the forearm so that the palm of the hand is facing upward.

Not all patients will be able to put each joint through a full range of motion. This is especially true of the elderly. As discussed in Chapter 4, calcium deposits in the joints, which accumulate during the aging process, limit the ability of the joint to function. Prolonged confinement in bed further compounds this problem unless exercises are performed to maintain the existing joint function.

There are three types of exercise, the appropriate type depending on the amount of assistance the patient requires to perform the range of motion. In passive exercises the nurse moves the patient's arm, leg, etc., through the range of motion. The patient does not move the body part himself, hence the term, "passive." In active assistive the nurse helps the patient move the joints through the range of motion. Active exercises are performed by the patient without help.

The patient starts range-of-motion exercises as soon as the physician indicates that he is medically able to do so. A program that is suited to the individual needs of the patient is developed. The doctor and the rehabilitation team discuss the patient's progress in achieving the set goals and formulate ways in which each team member can contribute to the attainment of these goals. Assisting the patient through range-of-motion exercises is not the responsibility of the physical therapist alone. The therapist may teach the nurse or other health worker how to perform the range-of-motion exercises geared to the particular patient's needs. If the exercises are not carried out in the patient unit as well as in physical therapy, the patient's progress will be hampered. The patient's joints are moved during the bed bath, and this is an excellent time to perform the prescribed range-of-motion exercises.

The patient and his family must understand why the exercises are being performed. Some family members may be alarmed that the nurse is forcing the patient to move when, in their opinion, the staff is there to perform all services. "The patient is there to rest and not to be disturbed by silly exercises." Once the rehabilitation team has gained the confidence of the patient and his family, the family members may be taught how to per-

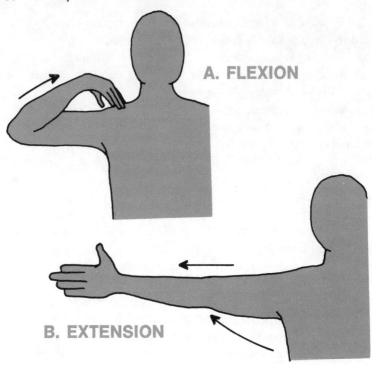

A. FLEXION

B. EXTENSION

C. INTERNAL ROTATION

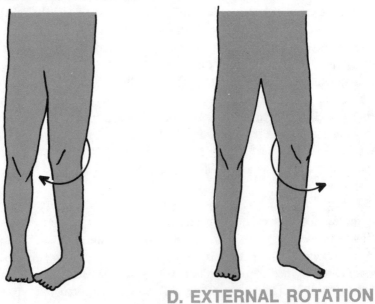

D. EXTERNAL ROTATION

Figure 6-1: Range of motion exercises.

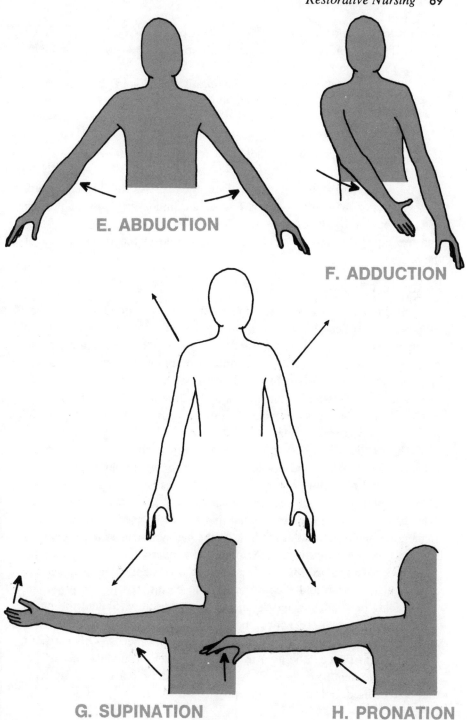

E. ABDUCTION

F. ADDUCTION

G. SUPINATION

H. PRONATION

form range-of-motion exercises. The following points should be emphasized:

1. The extremity should be held at the joint area, not at the fleshy part of the arm or leg.
2. The extremity should be grasped firmly but without undue pressure.
3. Exercises should not be done too quickly or with jerky motions.
4. The existing range of motion should be known, and care should be taken not to exceed this range, which would cause pain.
5. Each passive exercise should be repeated three times for an adequate effect.
6. At the first sign of patient fatigue, the exercise should be stopped.

Prevention of contractures is one of the important goals of nursing care. Through diligent, day-to-day adherence to the plan for range-of-motion exercises, the nurse can perform a vital role in the rehabilitation of the patient.

Prevention of Deformity

How many times have we seen the elderly person curled up in a favorite position in bed? No one is disturbed, for we know that after the nap or night's sleep, he will be "up and at it again." However, for the patient who is confined to bed, this favorite position can be a dangerous one. Although the position is comfortable, flexed arms, legs, and trunk will contribute to stiff joints and result in flexion contractures. Measures must be instituted immediately to provide the greatest possibility of returning the patient to his maximum potential.

The standard bed should be equipped with a firm mattress. A board between the mattress and springs will provide additional support. The patient should maintain proper body alignment as well as possible. Simple devices that will help the patient maintain proper alignment are readily available to the nurse. One of the first that should be used is the footboard. Remember, the footboard at the base of the bed is worthless if the patient's feet are 6 inches away from it. A footboard properly used is indicated for patients confined to bed for a period of time. This is a nursing care measure to prevent foot drop and should not have to be ordered by the physician. The nursing personnel should assume this responsibility. Should the physician have to write an order for a footboard or bed cradle, the nursing care team has been negligent in assessing the patient's needs. Other readily available items that can be used to assist the patient in maintaining proper alignment are sandbags and pillows. Splints and braces of various types may also be used, but they require a physician's order.

For patients who are totally disabled and depend on the nursing personnel to change their bed positions, a plan must be devised for turning. The patient's position in bed should be changed frequently—at least every two hours. The care plan indicates the time intervals between turning. Special types of beds, such as Stryker Frames and CircOlectric beds, may be used.

Prevention of Respiratory Complications

The reduced capacity to cough causing diminished elimination of secretions is a real problem for those elderly patients who are confined to bed. The threat of hypostatic pneumonia is ever-present. This is a condition in which there is a stagnation of blood at the bases of the lungs causing congestion to occur. Secretions accumulate due to prolonged immobility. These become thickened and difficult to expel due to inadequate fluid intake, certain kinds of drugs, and physiological changes associated with the aging process. Pathogenic organisms take advantage of the ideal growth media.

Initial symptoms may include slight elevations in the patient's vital signs. However, they may go unnoticed until marked difficulty in breathing occurs. If symptoms are not treated and the condition progresses, the outcome may be fatal. Therefore, it is essential that the nurse employ those principles of restorative nursing which will prevent hypostatic pneumonia. The nursing care plan should provide for daily deep breathing exercises for all immobilized patients in order to fully aerate the bases of the lungs and improve gaseous exchange in the alveoli. The patient should be moved into a position that will promote ease in breathing and allow for lung expansion. The physician may order intermittent positive pressure breathing treatments. This procedure is discussed in Chapter 10.

Frequent turning will aid the patient to loosen and expel thick mucous secretions. The nurse must teach and encourage the patient to cough deeply and at frequent intervals. The patient should be instructed to inhale deeply several times and then cough forcibly into two tissues. Shallow coughs are useless because they will not facilitate the removal of mucous from the lower lung. Patients who have severe respiratory difficulty may benefit from postural drainage to remove thickened secretions.

Prevention of Decubitus Ulcers

The patient who is confined to bed and unable to move himself is most susceptible to decubitus ulcers. In addition to immobility, other factors that contribute to skin breakdown are poor nutrition, severe debilitation from prolonged illness, excess weight or being underweight, and urinary and fecal incontinence.

Several measures can be taken to prevent the development of skin breakdown. Frequent moving, turning, and positioning of the patient can reduce prolonged pressure on the skin. Those sites that are particularly susceptible to this problem should be inspected when the patient is turned. Areas to be observed include the bony prominences, such as the heels, ankles, hips, sacrum, shoulder blades, shoulders, and elbows; soft tissue pressure points, including the ears, abdomen, breasts, and buttocks; and the forehead, nose, back of the head, and areas beneath pendulous breasts. Any signs of redness should be reported promptly. The physician will order special ointments or devices to treat the problem and prevent skin breakdown.

Scrupulous skin care is essential for all bedridden patients. This includes washing with soap and water and drying the area well. Application of powder may be indicated in some areas. Lotion may be applied to very dry skin. At no time should creams or lotions be vigorously rubbed into the skin because the massaging of legs and arms may cause thrombi to be dislodged from a distal blood vessel. Thrombus formation may readily occur in the bedfast elderly patient.

Incontinence poses special problems in the prevention of decubitus because excreta is irritating to the skin and predisposes it to breakdown. After each elimination the skin should be washed and dried thoroughly. Soiled linens and linen protectors should be changed. The bottom bed clothing should be free of wrinkles. If some type of diaper or protective pants is used, it should be checked at the time of turning and changed if necessary. Cleansing of the skin accompanies the changing procedure.

The doctor may order special devices that help to prevent pressure sores, including sheepskin and protectors for heels and elbows. The sheepskin will not be of any value unless the patient's skin is directly upon the device. Since it is difficult to keep a patient clean if he is incontinent, two sheepskins may be needed—one to wash and one to wear. Keep the cost of the sheepskin in mind when ordering two.

Air mattresses are also used to prevent decubitus formation. The inflated mattress should not be completely filled with air, but should have some slack so that it will give to accommodate the body weight. Never pin anything to the bottom bedding because you might puncture the mattress and cause it to deflate.

The alternating pressure pad is similar to the air mattress in that it too is made of heavy-duty plastic and contains many small compartments. These chambers fill and empty with air, thereby providing a massagelike action against the body surface. Be certain that the tubes leading from the pad to the motor are connected correctly.

The water bed has been used most effectively to prevent skin breakdown. The manufacturer's instructions for filling the bed and applying linens should be followed carefully. Small water-filled pads may be used as sit-upons to prevent pressure and to allow comfort. These pads are especially useful for the patient in a wheelchair.

Devices such as donuts and air rings are frowned upon, since they only cause pressure and have no therapeutic or preventive value.

Providing Adequate Nutrition

Another important factor related to the prevention of deformities and pressure sores is the maintenance of an adequate nutritional state for the patient. The old cliché "you are what you eat" is not fiction. Upon admission to the health care facility, the patient's nutritional status is assessed, and an appropriate diet is ordered.

A few factors contributing to a patient's poor state of nutrition may be the length of time he has had the disease, limited income and his reliance on bulky, inexpensive carbohydrate foods rather than protein, and poor or no teeth. No matter what the cause of poor nutrition, the goal is clear— to help the patient achieve an optimum nutritional level.

In addition to a balanced diet, including the four basic food groups, the patient confined to bed requires increased amounts of proteins. As mentioned previously, muscles need protein for proper functioning. When the body is inactive over a period of time, some protein is lost, and muscle weakness occurs. Therefore, increased amounts of protein should be added to the diet to counterbalance the loss and hopefully reduce muscle weakness. Foods high in calcium content are contraindicated for the elderly person who is confined to bed for a period of time, because the incidence of formation of renal calculi is greatly increased. For this reason milk and milk products should be used in minimal quantities.

Because of the patient's physical inactivity, the physician will want to make sure that sufficient roughage is included in his diet. The lower intestinal tract tends to become sluggish; roughage stimulates peristaltic action, thereby reducing problems of elimination. Daily fluid intake of approximately 2,000 cc may also be indicated. Normal functioning of the urinary and digestive systems is of the utmost importance. The diet can contribute greatly to the prevention of complications, which delay the start of the active rehabilitation process.

The overweight patient may present a real problem to the rehabilitation team. Initiation of an effective weight-reduction program may be prescribed as the first step in the whole process of rehabilitation. The patient can ill afford to compound his problem by carrying excess weight. If active rehabilitation is to take place, the body must be prepared to assume an active role.

The bedfast patient's highest energy level usually occurs in the morning. As the day progresses, his stamina decreases. Because of this the best meal of the day may be breakfast. For this reason the dietitian may plan a large meal for breakfast, with lunch running second in size, and the evening meal being the smallest of the day. Thus, the patient's fatigue and low energy levels in the evening are taken into consideration.

The patient who can feed himself will rely on the staff to provide an atmosphere conducive to eating. He also depends on the staff to place the tray so that it is not beyond his reach. There is nothing worse than being hungry and not being able to get near enough to the food to eat. Attractive trays, with the hot foods hot and the cold foods cold, help to enhance the patient's appetite.

The patient may require a long period of time to finish his meal, and the nurse should be sure he has enough time. Following the removal of the tray, she should note the patient's intake. Were certain foods untouched? A high-protein diet is of no use if the meat is left sitting on the plate. The nurse should inquire about the reasons for a patient's not eating certain foods and relay this information via the charge nurse to the dietitian so that the menu can be adjusted.

Some patients who are able to feed themselves may require some assistance from the staff. The nursing care plan should spell out the amount and type of assistance required—cutting food, buttering the bread, pouring liquids, etc. It is the nursing personnel's responsibility to see that the patient requiring assistance receives it immediately upon the arrival of the tray. This eases patient frustration and allows the additional time needed to complete the meal. For those whose physical disability makes it difficult or impossible for them to eat with regular utensils, several self-help devices, such as built-up handles on spoons and forks, plate guards, and combination knife and fork, can be used. (See Figure 6-2.)

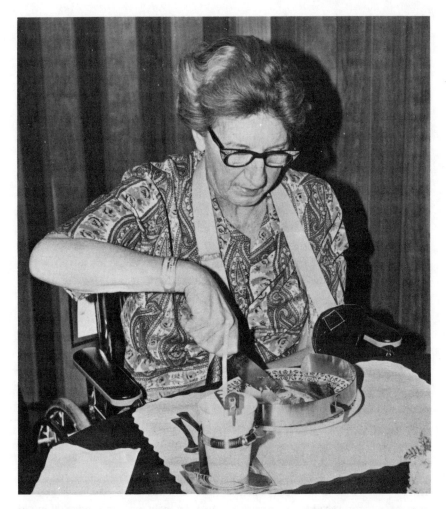

Figure 6-2: Special devices aid the stroke patient at mealtime. Note plate guard, rocker knife, and universal holder on cup.

Patients who are totally dependent on the staff for their food intake may find mealtime one of the most frustrating parts of the day. To have to rely on others for this basic simple activity can be a humiliating experience. The way in which the staff handles meals can either contribute to the rehabilitation process or retard it. The nurse must have adequate time to help the patient, and in turn, the patient must be given adequate time for eating.

Mealtime is also a social time, and the socializing aspect should not be neglected because "it takes up too much time." Family members who are able to visit at mealtime may provide the social atmosphere so conducive to eating, and they may assist in feeding the patient his lunch or dinner. They may also provide information regarding the patient's eating habits, thereby giving clues to ways in which the nurse can individualize the mealtime.

The nursing care plan should indicate all modifications in mealtime practices so that all personnel caring for the patient are knowledgeable and can implement the plan. As the patient assumes more responsibility for his dietary intake, the care plan should be modified and updated. Supplemental feedings during the day and evening may be ordered in the form of nourishing liquids. These contribute to the total fluid intake. The entire nursing staff, acting as a team, assumes responsibility for seeing that adequate amounts of fluids are given to the elderly patient. Also, it takes such a short time to stop and chat for a few minutes while assisting the patient with his fruit juice or soup. Providing adequate nutrition prepares the way for the time when active rehabilitation takes place.

Providing for Elimination

Elimination from both the bowel and the bladder can cause problems for the bedfast patient. Constipation frequently results from lack of exercise, insufficient fluids, and inadequate roughage in the diet. The patient's fluid intake should be recorded so that all personnel will be aware of his need for liquids. Many times the patient can be taught to record his own intake, and this will help him to realize how much he needs to drink each day.

It is important for the patient to establish regular bowel habits. Since most people feel the desire to evacuate following meals (especially breakfast), this would be an appropriate time to offer the bedpan. Make the patient as comfortable as possible, provide privacy, and have the call button within reach. Do not leave the patient sitting on the bedpan too long; check with him after ten minutes. If he has been unable to defecate, remove the pan and offer it at a later time. Nursing personnel must observe and record the stools accurately. There is no excuse for not knowing if the patient has had a bowel movement. He cannot manage to evacuate without someone's assistance, and the results must be charted.

When constipation occurs, the physician may order suppositories— glycerine or medicated. These are generally as effective as the cleansing enema and are more acceptable to the patient. If constipation is not corrected, the patient may develop a fecal impaction. The professional nurse or the licensed practical nurse should check the patient for an impaction and remove it if possible. Since this procedure is very uncomfortable, all efforts should be made to have the patient maintain normal bowel function.

The elderly are very sensitive and embarrassed about incontinence. Many times they are so humiliated about having an accident in bed that they will not tell anyone about it. Nursing personnel must be kind, understanding, and above all alert to this situation. Certainly, if the patient is being positioned every two hours, his output could be checked at this time. Cerebral vascular accident, severe confusion, or senility may cause the patient to be unaware of his incontinence or unable to ask for assistance. The nursing staff must be alert to the problems of this patient and quick to meet his needs in order to prevent skin problems. Urinary incontinence may be caused by the patient's disease condition, his having to wait too long for the bedpan or urinal (especially at night), or his inability to void in an unnatural position. Nursing care personnel should offer the bedpan frequently and at those times when the patient is most likely to void—immediately upon awakening, before and after meals, before bathing, and upon retiring. If the older person is restless during the night, the bedpan should be offered to him, since nocturia is common.

If these measures are not successful, the physician may order the use of special devices such as the plastic sheath and bag for the incontinent male or diaperlike protective panties for women. If incontinence occurs only during the sleeping hours, fluids might be withheld during the evening, and a program of bedtime voiding instituted. In addition, the patient may use protective plastic pants during the night.

A retention catheter may be ordered for some patients who have a problem with urinary incontinence. Such a device will keep the patient dry, but its use is discouraged, since it may cause urinary tract infection. Therefore, the indwelling catheter is used as a last resort in the treatment of incontinence. Special care must be taken to ensure sterility of the catheter's drainage system. Tubing should be checked for kinks; the collection bag should be emptied at the end of each shift; and the amount, color, and consistency of the urine should be reported and recorded. Catheter irrigation is ordered by the physician. It is an aseptic procedure, and the equipment and solution must be sterile.

The doctor may order the indwelling catheter to be clamped for four hours and then unclamped to allow the bladder to empty. In addition, the catheter may be clamped while the patient sleeps. The drainage system is clamped and opened at specified intervals to allow the bladder to fill and empty in a way that approximates normal voiding. This is done to prepare for the removal of the catheter. Once it has been removed, the patient care team must check carefully to make sure the patient is voiding adequate quantities. Urinary output must be measured and recorded accurately.

Many elderly patients experience urinary retention. This may be the result of a disease condition, but often it is caused by the patient's inability to void in an unnatural position. Nursing measures to stimulate voiding, such as providing a warm bedpan or pouring warm water over genitalia, should be utilized. Usually the problem is corrected when the patient is able to use the toilet or commode.

Bowel and bladder training may be indicated for some patients. The rehabilitation team will evaluate the patient's readiness for such training. The training procedure is carried out by a professional nurse who is a clinical specialist in rehabilitation nursing and by the physical therapist.

Helping the Patient to Acquire Relative Independence

How independent can one become if he is confined to bed? Independence can be measured by the number of activities the patient can perform without assistance. Moving and turning in bed are prerequisites to assuming an upright position and ambulation. Self-feeding has already been discussed. The staff, however, must perform preliminary tasks that will enable the patient to assume some independence. For example, the patient must have the tray served to him before he can feed himself.

The nurse participates in the rehabilitation process by encouraging patient activities that foster independence. As stated previously, the goal of rehabilitation is to return the patient to his optimum level of functioning. Steps toward this goal include the patient's beginning performance of self-care tasks while he is confined to bed. Self-care activities include those that are performed in the course of each day. They are routines so well established that the healthy person performs them almost without thinking, and include washing the face and hands, brushing teeth, combing hair, shaving, and using the toilet. Such routine tasks are called activities of daily living, or ADL. Before the patient can begin to perform these activities of daily living, he must be able to use muscles and joints and have sufficient strength. Range-of-motion exercises are the forerunners to the successful performance of ADL. When the patient performs these activities, two main objectives are being accomplished: (1) his muscles and joints are being actively exercised and strengthened and (2) his morale is lifted. When the patient is able to sit in an upright position, he will be able to assume more responsibility for self-care. His activities should begin with simple tasks and progress to the more difficult ones. To the nurse, the time it takes the patient to wash his face without assistance may seem like an eternity, and his face may not be as clean as we would like. But, nevertheless, the patient's washing his face marks the beginning of his independence. Each small step must be encouraged by the rehabilitation team. Doing for the patient when he can do for himself is a monumental error, which everyone on the team must guard against. The progress of the patient in ADL must be communicated to all members of the nursing staff. One method, in addition to verbal communication, is through the patient care plan. The family must also be informed of the patient's progress and given the reasons for encouraging self-help, so that the family will support and encourage ADL during visits.

STUDY QUESTIONS AND PROBLEMS

1. What provisions for restorative nursing exist in the nursing homes you have visited?
2. Observe a bed bath. Note the kinds of movements that the patient's joints undergo during this procedure.
3. The father of a friend of yours will be discharged from the hospital next week and will be confined to bed. The family has asked you to assist them in finding inexpensive materials to make a foot board and cradle. What is your advice?
4. List some high-protein foods that could be offered as in-between meal feedings for the bedfast patient.

BIBLIOGRAPHY

A Handbook of Rehabilitative Nursing Techniques in Hemiplegia. Minneapolis: Kenny Rehabilitation Institute, 1964.

Anderson, Helen C. *Newton's Geriatric Nursing.* 5th ed. Saint Louis: C. V. Mosby, 1971.

Beland, Irene. *Clinical Nursing: Pathophysiological and Psychosocial Approaches.* 2nd ed. New York: Macmillan, 1970.

Carnevali, Doris, and Breuchner, Susan. "Immobilization: Reassessment of a Concept." *American Journal of Nursing,* July 1970, p. 1503.

Coles, Catherine, and Bergstrom, Doris. *Basic Positioning Procedures.* Minneapolis: Kenny Rehabilitation Institute, 1971.

Halley, Lydia. "The Physical Therapist—Who, What and How." *American Journal of Nursing,* July 1970, p .1521.

Hirschberg, Gerald G.; Lewis, Leon; and Thomas, Dorothy. *Rehabilitation: A Manual for the Care of the Disabled and Elderly.* Philadelphia: J. B. Lippincott, 1964.

Little, Dolores, and Carnevali, Doris. *Nursing Care Planning.* Philadelphia: J. B. Lippincott, 1969.

Martin, Nancy; King, Rosemarie; and Suchinski, Joyce. "The Nurse Therapist in a Rehabilitation Setting." *American Journal of Nursing,* August 1970, pp. 1694–1697.

Mitchell, Helen; Rynbergen, Henderika; Anderson, Linnea; and Dibble, Marjorie. *Cooper's Nutrition in Health and Disease.* 15th ed. Philadelphia: J. B. Lippincott, 1968.

Nursing Care of the Skin. Rehabilitation Publication, no. 711. Minneapolis: American Rehabilitation Foundation, 1967.

Olson, Edith, et al. "Hazards of Immobility." *American Journal of Nursing,* April 1967, p. 781.

Rossman, Isadore. *Clinical Geriatrics.* Philadelphia: J. B. Lippincott, 1968.

Sorenson, Lois, and Ulrich, Patricia. *Ambulation: A Manual for Nurses.* Rehabilitation Publication, no. 707. Minneapolis: American Rehabilitation Foundation, 1966.

Toohey, Patricia, and Larson, Corrine. *Range of Motion Exercise: Key to Joint Mobility.* Rehabilitation Publication, no. 703. Minneapolis: American Rehabilitation Foundation, 1968.

West, Wilma. "Occupational Therapy Philosophy and Perspective." *American Journal of Nursing,* August 1968, p. 1708.

Yates, Judith. *Moving and Lifting Patients: Principles and Techniques.* Minneapolis: Kenny Rehabilitation Institute, 1970.

7

Activities of Daily Living

"Oh, how I hate to get up in the morning," a line from a song, is also a feeling expressed by millions of workers as they prepare for the day's routine. However, the disabled, confined to bed, would gladly trade places with those who complain about these early morning tasks.

Self-care activities, which are taken for granted by the healthy adult, need to be relearned by the disabled. For many, this relearning is slow and painstaking. Just as the infant crawls before he walks, so too the handicapped person must master elementary activities of daily living before he can go on to the more complex. The patient has had to learn how to move around in bed. Rolling and turning, first with assistance and then independently, prepare him physically for assuming the sitting position. When he can sit upright, he is able to feed himself more easily and to perform other self-care activities, such as washing, shaving, and combing his hair. Members of the patient care team provide the foundation on which the rehabilitative process is built by instituting measures that help the patient to become ready to assume an active role.

Since the nursing team initially spends the largest amount of time with the patient, team members must take the opportunity to assist in motivating the patient to perform self-care activities. Unless the patient is motivated to achieve independence, the battle is lost. The nurse, then, acts as the stimulator, the encourager, the helper when needed. This is nursing in its most complete sense.

As the patient progresses in his self-care activities, special assistance from other health disciplines will be needed. Some transfer activities, for example, may be more easily learned when the patient is in the physical therapy unit. The physical therapist may teach the patient to perform certain exercises to strengthen muscle groups. The nursing team must know what the therapist has taught the patient so that he can be encouraged to practice the exercises properly. What goes on in the physical therapy department is vitally important to the patient's ultimate independence, and it is up to the nurse to see that continuity of care is maintained between his trips to the physical therapy unit.

The nursing personnel assumes a supportive role by reinforcing the specific competencies of other allied health workers. Those in one specialty cannot afford to be jealous of another's abilities in meeting the patient's needs—especially when his need is for independence.

The physical therapist is a specialist in the field of rehabilitation. Under the direction of the physician, he tests the patient's ability to perform self-care activities, teaches the patient techniques such as crutch walking, transfer activities, and wheelchair manipulation, and administers treatments necessary to restore maximum muscle function. The physical therapist's role includes instructing the patient's family and nursing personnel in the specific activities the patient should perform. The physical therapist's instructions should be clearly understood by everyone. The patient should not be given conflicting directions on how to crutch walk—one set of directions from the physical therapist and another from a health worker in the patient unit. Each team member must work in unison with the other. At conferences the rehabilitation team shares information regarding the patient's progress in self-care activities and discusses his attitudes and emotional reactions to the slow process of rehabilitation.

The occupational therapist also evaluates the patient's ability to perform tasks and develops a suitable program, taking into consideration the patient's likes and dislikes and occupational and recreational interests. For example, the elderly woman who will be confined to a wheelchair when she returns home must learn to function in the kitchen. The occupational therapist works with her so that, if possible, she will achieve independence. Through the development of recreational skills, her eye-hand coordination may be strengthened, and at the same time the activity provides an interesting recreational outlet. The primary purpose, however, of all activities is therapeutic. Teaching is a major function of the occupational therapist. The family, as well as the members of the rehabilitation team, must be aware of the instructions the patient receives in this department.

As the patient progresses toward his maximum potential, the physician, as head of the rehabilitation team, orders changes in the physical therapy, occupational therapy, and nursing care regimens. Each discipline has its limitations. Only when everyone works together can progress toward independence be achieved.

MOBILITY IN BED

The patient's mobility in bed, assisted or unassisted, is a prerequisite to his assuming a sitting position. The purposes of moving the patient in bed are: (1) to prevent the complications of enforced bedrest, (2) to stimulate and encourage the patient psychologically, and (3) to enable the patient to become actively involved in the activities of daily living and thus to begin the rehabilitation process.

There are several methods for helping the patient to move in bed. One technique is that of muscle-training exercises taught by the physical therapist. However, these exercises are not usually appropriate for the elderly disabled, because the physical demands are too rigorous.

Another method would be the use of appliances that assist the patient in moving. Bed rails will help him to turn. A trapeze or some kind of a pull-up device attached to the foot of the bed may help him to sit upright. (See Figure 7-1.)

Passive positioning of the patient will also aid in increasing his mobility. Perhaps the patient cannot sit up from the dorsal recumbent position. If the nurse elevates the back of the bed (passive positioning), the patient may be able to grasp the side rails and sit up.

The technique selected to increase the patient's mobility while he is still bedfast depends on his physical strength, his progress toward recovery, his limitations, and his abilities. The nursing team, the physical therapist, and the physician will cooperate in the planning and institution of procedures preparatory to getting the patient up and sitting out of bed.

When the patient is elevated to a sitting position for the first time, it is important to watch for untoward reactions. Dizziness and fainting, caused by hypotension, are not uncommon, especially when the individual has been bedfast for a prolonged period. For this reason the patient should be gradually eased into a full sitting position. Each day the head of the bed may be raised slightly higher until the patient becomes physically adjusted to sitting upright.

Dangling (sitting the patient on the side of the bed while his legs and feet dangle) is an old method of preparing the patient to sit in a chair. This practice is generally frowned on because it places excess pressure on

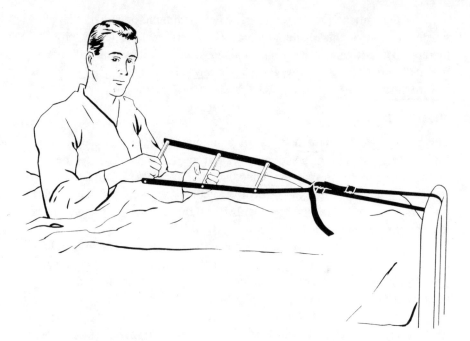

Figure 7-1: Pull-up device, "Patient Aid." *(Rehabilitation Products: J. T. Posey Co.)*

the back of the legs and is thought to be a contributing factor in the development of thrombi. Dangling can be dangerous if the bed is elevated to full height, since the patient is liable to fall. If the bed can be lowered so that the patient's feet are firmly on the floor and the overbed table can be placed across his lap, a few minutes in this position may be permitted, but this should not be maintained for a lengthy period, because the patient will develop dependent edema of the lower limbs. Also, as discussed previously, complications may occur when any position is maintained for a prolonged length of time.

When the patient is physically able to get out of bed, it is important that he understand exactly what is going to happen. The nurse must carefully explain each step of the procedure to the patient in order to gain his confidence and cooperation. The elderly disabled person may be very reluctant to get out of bed for fear of falling and injuring himself. The reassurance given by the nurse together with competent management will help to allay the patient's fears. The nursing care team will formulate a plan for the transfer from bed to chair. The patient's abilities are of primary consideration in this plan. The health care team will assess the patient's physiological condition by observing his physical reaction to increased activity. Other factors of importance in the development of the plan include the patient's joint mobility, strength, endurance, and balance. The patient's comprehension is another essential consideration. If he has difficulty understanding and following verbal instructions, it is important to use simple directions and to set up a consistent transfer routine.

TRANSFERS

There are several methods of transfer: standing, sitting, and lifting. If a standing transfer is selected, the patient must be able to bear weight on one or both legs. In addition, he needs strength in his arms and the ability to maintain balance. Sitting transfers are utilized for patients such as those with a bilateral amputation or paralysis of both lower limbs, who cannot balance and support weight on the lower limbs. Transfer by lifting is accomplished by moving the patient manually or by using a mechanical lift. Transfer by a mechanical lift is indicated for the patient who cannot move independently and cannot be moved by one or two persons. The severely debilitated patient or one with advanced cardiac problems may be transferred in this manner. The method is safe and efficient, and prevents strain on both the patient and personnel. The patient does not take an active role in the procedure, but sitting up will help to increase his general mobility.

The selection and placement of equipment is vital for a safe and effective transfer. The bed must be lowered so that the top surface of the mattress is even with the seat of the chair. Usually, the patient is transferred into a wheelchair. If another type of chair is to be used, it should have a straight back and armrests, and should provide comfort and proper support. (See Figure 7-2.)

Numerous types of wheelchairs and special features are available. A wheelchair can be custom-ordered for the patient and include such features as removable armrests, reclining backs, and extended brake pedals. It may be self-propelled or driven by an electric motor. The physician and the rehabilitation team will determine what special features are to be ordered. These will depend on the patient's physical condition and the plan for rehabilitation.

The following suggestions will aid in effecting transfers: Keep the transfer surfaces as close to each other as possible. If half-length side rails are available, they will assist the patient both in sitting up and in supporting himself while sitting. If they are not available, provide firm hand support. Place the equipment so that it meets the patient's needs. For example, if the patient has hemiplegia, place the wheelchair alongside the bed on the patient's uninvolved side.

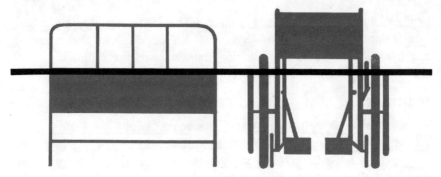

Figure 7-2: Transfer surfaces of equal heights. *(American Rehabilitation Foundation)*

Most times the patient will require assistance with the standing transfer. Only the essential help should be given. He should do as much for himself as possible. But be certain that he has adequate protection from falls.

Good body mechanics are important in assuring safety for both the patient and the nurse. When preparing for the transfer, the nurse should stand close to the patient and keep her feet apart, with one foot slightly ahead of the other, in order to provide a good base of support. Assistance should be provided by placing one's arms around the patient's waist. In some instances a transfer belt may be buckled firmly around the patient's waist so that it can be grasped during the transfer procedure. Lifting should be done with the long strong muscles of the legs. The assistant should bend her knees, lower her hips, and help the patient to a standing position by straightening these joints. The patient should be able to see the seat of the chair. If the equipment is positioned properly, the assistant shifts her weight from one foot to another to accomplish the transfer.

In most instances the nursing team will schedule the transfer activity for the morning hours. The patient has more energy and stamina at this time. If the patient is an arthritic who experiences joint stiffness upon awakening, the transfer should be scheduled for later in the day, when his joints are less painful.

The following procedure may be utilized for the standing, or weight-bearing, transfer:

1. Explain the procedure to the patient.
2. Bring all equipment to the room.
3. Lower the bed so that the mattress is the same height as the seat of the wheelchair.
4. Position the wheelchair at a slight angle to the bed so that it is facing the foot of the bed.

5. Lock bed wheels and wheelchair brakes. Position footrests so they are out of the way.
6. Bring the patient to sitting position.
7. Help the patient to swing his legs over the edge of the mattress so that he is sitting erect on the side of the bed.
8. Put on the patient's robe, shoes, and socks.
9. Stand directly in front of the patient with your feet slightly apart. Bend hips and knees so that you are level with the patient.
10. Place your arms around the patient's waist. Clasp one hand over the other wrist behind the patient's back. Straighten hips and

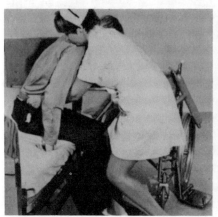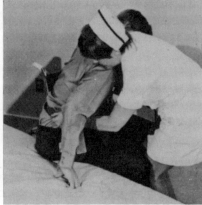

Figure 7-3: Assisted sitting transfer. *(American Rehabilitation Foundation)* Standing in front of the patient with feet slightly apart, the assistant bends her hips and

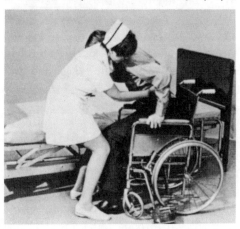

knees to lower herself to the patient's level. She grips the transfer belt and assists him in angling his hips toward the chair, and also in positioning his hands and feet as needed. To prevent the patient from sliding forward, she supports his knees with hers. Using the transfer belt, she assists in lifting his buttocks while allowing him to see the surface to which he is transferring. Throughout the transfer she must allow the patient to lean forward so he can maintain trunk balance. She then helps him to move back in the chair by pushing her knees against his.

knees and raise the patient to a standing position. You may lock your knees against the patient's to provide additional support and prevent the patient's knees from buckling.

11. Stand close to the patient and help him to pivot so that the new sitting surface is directly behind his legs.

12. Have the patient place his hands on the wheelchair arms and slowly lower himself into the sitting position. Give assistance as necessary.

The procedure is reversed when assisting the patient to return to bed.

The sitting transfer may be achieved by one of several techniques. With the push-up method the patient raises himself up with his arms as he transfers from bed to chair. If a trapeze is available, the pull-up or chinning method may be used. For the pull-up sitting transfer the patient must have strong arm muscles and the stamina to pull himself up and swing from one surface to the other.

Perhaps with the elderly the most useful technique for a sitting transfer is to use a sliding board as a bridge between the two transfer surfaces. The patient still has to push himself up to move along the board, but the nursing personnel can render any necessary assistance. (See Figure 7-4.)

The patient should perform the activities of daily living, such as eating, washing, and brushing the teeth, when he is in the wheelchair. The patient's responsibility for ADL should be increased as the length of time he is out of bed increases. Initially, it will be sufficient to transfer the patient to the chair, since the procedure will be very tiring. The patient should be permitted to rest in the chair for a short period and returned to bed before he becomes fatigued.

Once the patient is accustomed to sitting out of bed, he may be taught to propel the wheelchair about his room, in and out of the bathroom, and down the hall. Special problems in maneuvering the wheelchair will be dealt with in the physical therapy department.

PERSONAL HYGIENE

Now that the patient is in a wheelchair, his environment can be changed. No longer is the patient's activity confined to the immediate vicinity of his bed. The bathroom and shower area, once out of bounds, are now within reach. Gaining independence in one's toilet habits and other personal hygiene routines is most important to all patients. They should be shown how to maneuver the wheelchair into the bathroom and transfer to the toilet, shower, or tub. The physical therapist will consider the patient's physical ability, his disease condition, and other pertinent information, and instruct the patient in the proper transfer technique.

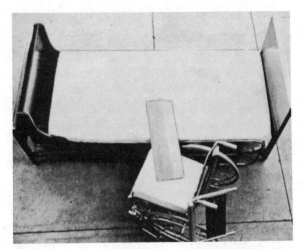

Figure 7-4: Sliding board placement. *(American Rehabilitation Foundation)*

If the patient's physical condition so warrants, the rehabilitation team may suggest the use of a bedside commode as a first step toward independence. Usually, the patient adjusts quite easily to using the commode, since he uses it in a more natural position than the bedpan. Elimination problems lessen when the patient is permitted out of bed to use the commode. The same transfer procedure is used to move the patient to the commode that is used to get him from the bed to the wheelchair. Toilet tissue and the call light cord must be within easy reach of the patient.

Certain modifications in the bathroom area are necessary so that easy, safe transfers to and from the wheelchair can be accomplished. Grab bars or handrails on the wall beside the toilet or right-angle rails bolted to the wall and floor will help the patient in transferring. As explained previously, transfer surfaces must be the same height if the transfer is to be accomplished easily. Thus, the wheelchair seat and the toilet seat should be the same height. The average toilet seat is about 16 inches from the floor, which is considerably lower than the wheelchair, but many health care facilities have installed toilets that are about 20 inches from the floor to aid patients in making wheelchair to toilet transfers. Raised toilet seats may be obtained from hospital supply companies. These are attached to the regular toilet (preferably to the toilet bowl) and provide the proper seat height. If the patient has difficulty maintaining balance, his clothing may need to be adjusted while he is in the wheelchair, both before and after the transfer to the toilet. A zipper in the backrest of the wheelchair will permit patients who are unable to assume a standing position to slide backwards onto the toilet seat. (See Figure 7-5.)

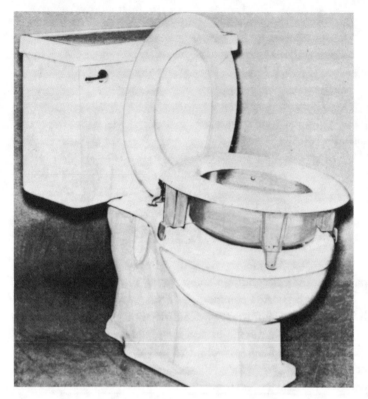

Figure 7-5: Portable raised toilet seat with shield. *(Hirschberg, Lewis, and Thomas, Rehabilitation: A Manual for the Care of the Disabled and Elderly)*

Performing routine personal hygiene activities at the sink is not usually as complicated. The patient looks forward to taking a sponge bath at the sink after receiving bed baths for a period of time. In order for the patient to be as close as possible to the sink, wheelchair armrests need to be removed. Adjustments in the bathroom will also need to be made. For example, towel racks, shelves for keeping oral hygiene supplies, and the soap dish should be within easy reach of the wheelchair patient, and the mirror over the sink needs to be low enough for the patient to benefit from it. Some patients may initially prefer to use a lapboard, which rests on top of the armrests of the wheelchair, when washing. Water basin, soap, and personal hygiene equipment are placed on the lapboard for the patient's use.

Elderly women should be encouraged to apply cosmetics if they were accustomed to using them before hospitalization. This gives the necessary boost to the morale. Every lady likes to look her best. In the extended care facility there is often a barber or beautician whose services can be called upon. The wheelchair patient can take advantage of these services more easily.

Although performing daily personal hygiene tasks at the bathroom sink is a psychological improvement over being bathed in bed, the patient looks forward to being able to take his own shower or tub bath. The physical therapist instructs the patient regarding bathtub and/or shower transfers. Newer rehabilitation centers have wheelchair shower rooms, where the patient takes a shower while seated in the wheelchair, thus no transfer activity is required. Patients using a regular shower stall are transferred from the wheelchair to a bench or chair installed in the shower. In order to prevent the chair or bench from slipping, rubber suction tips are attached to its legs. Strips of safety-tread tape are applied to the floor. In addition, rubber mats need to be placed on the floor of the shower to prevent slipping. Grab bars within easy reach of the patient assist in safe transfer and maintenance of the patient's balance. A shampoo hose should be connected to the shower head so that the patient can regulate the direction of the spray as well as the temperature of the water. The patient may find a long-handled brush most useful for getting at hard-to-reach areas of the back and legs. If the soap is hung on a rope around the patient's neck, it cannot slip out of his reach—a safety hazard as well as a frustrating experience.

The most difficult transfer is that from the wheelchair to a bathtub and back. The patient should first practice the procedure without water and under the guidance and supervision of the physical therapist. Grab bars, handrails, and strips of safety-tread tape in the bottom and on the rim of the tub are all essential for safe transfers. The patient usually transfers from the wheelchair to a chair placed in the bathtub and then to a lower seat within the tub.

Because the time it takes to complete a shower or bath is prolonged, the less rushed evening hours may be the most appropriate time for the patient to accomplish this task. With trips to physical therapy, occupational therapy, speech therapy and so on, the daylight hours are crammed with activity. The patient's rushing to take a bath or shower may contribute to a serious accident, negating any progress made in rehabilitation. The nursing care team needs to plan, with the patient, a realistic schedule that meets the patient's personal hygiene needs. The morning bath or shower may not be the answer; flexibility is.

CLOTHING AND DRESSING

The selection of clothing for the patient is based on his physical limitations and planned activities. When a patient can sit up out of bed in street clothing, he will feel that he is on the road to recovery.

If the patient is to dress himself, he must have good sitting balance and the ability to use at least one arm. He will put on most of his clothes while sitting on the side of the bed. He can lie down to pull up his trousers.

Clothing should be washable and loose-fitting, and it should open at the front or side. Zippers, buttons, and ties that open in the back of a garment present difficulties even for the nonhandicapped person, and this type of clothing should be avoided.

Slacks are recommended for both men and women, because they are easy to put on and will prevent exposure during therapy. Sometimes elderly women will object to wearing pants, which is understandable, since they are not accustomed to this kind of apparel. They need to understand the reasons for wearing such clothing. Once they experience the comfort and warmth that these garments provide, most women readily accept the idea.

Sometimes garments need to be altered to allow for ease in dressing. Tabs or rings may be added to zippers; buttonholes may be enlarged to accommodate larger buttons; and buttons may be sewed on with elastic thread. Velcro strips may be substituted for other types of fasteners. Brassieres present a vexing problem for handicapped women. Bras with front closures may be used, or the standard bra may be hooked in the front and then turned around to the back. The arms are then placed through the straps.

Shoes should provide good support for the foot and have a low heel to ensure good balance. Oxfords are recommended. Socks should have a loosely fitted top and be easy to pull on. At first the patient will need help putting on his shoes and socks. Tying the laces will be a frustrating task for the patient who has the use of only one arm. Elastic laces and long-handled shoehorns will make it easier for the patient to put on his shoes.

When the patient is ready to dress, the pieces of clothing should be placed within his reach in the order in which he will put them on, and the nurse should provide encouragement and assistance as needed.

EATING ACTIVITIES

Eating may be one of the first activities that the patient attempts. As soon as he is able to sit out of bed for thirty to sixty minutes, he should eat one meal sitting up.

The tray should be placed on the overbed table, and the patient should be given assistance when necessary. Gradually, the nursing staff will give the patient less and less help as he learns to feed himself. The occupational therapist will teach the patient new methods of cutting food, buttering bread, drinking, etc. Devices that can be used to make self-feeding easier include plate guards that help the patient to get the food onto his fork and to keep the food from sliding off the plate, suction cups that firmly anchor dishes and prevent slipping, a knife-fork that combines both utensils into one, and a nontippable cup that prevents spilling.

As soon as possible the patient should eat in the group dining area. Eating in the dining room will provide an opportunity for him to have social contact with others. Also, he will become aware of the importance of eating habits that are acceptable to others at the table. If a dining room is not available, a table in the lounge or sun porch may be set up for dining. Whenever possible, the patient should not dine alone. Dining alone can be very depressing. It is almost enough to take the appetite away.

DIVERSIONAL ACTIVITIES

Many health care facilities have well-planned recreational activities, some under the direction of the occupational therapy department or a volunteer auxiliary association. Unfortunately, however, many nursing homes and extended care facilities provide few recreational opportunities. The blaring television set in the dayroom may be the only means of recreation other than visits from family and relatives. The nurse needs to assist the patient in satisfying his requirements for diversion and recreation.

The occupational therapist and/or nurse should help to stimulate the patient's participation in nongroup activities, the particular activity depending on the patient's likes and dislikes and his physical and mental abilities. Examples of such activities include reading books and magazines, doing various kinds of puzzles, knitting, crocheting, handicraft activities, playing various musical instruments, and painting. Some patients may be interested in planning group activities along with the staff of the health care facility. A favorite activity is bingo—it has a quality of being a group activity although the patient can still maintain his independence while playing the game. Mah-Jong and card games, especially pinochle, are also favorites. Discussion groups for those sharing similar interests and concerns help the elderly to maintain intellectual stimulation as well as recreation. In addition to offering spiritual consolation, religious services also have an element of diversion—enabling the patient to sing hymns and participate in the service.

Seasonal parties on such occasions as Christmas, Chanukah, Easter, and Independence Day, usually sponsored by community churches or religious groups, also provide an opportunity for patients to socialize with other patients, staff members, and members of the community. Unfortunately, parties of this nature usually occur only a few times during the year. For the most part, it is the staff that is responsible for providing day-to-day recreational and diversional outlets for patients.

Perhaps one of the biggest contributions the staff can make to the patient's diversional therapy is to encourage him to get out of doors. The patient's activities need not be confined to a room inside. Perhaps the patient cannot propel his wheelchair by himself and has to rely on the staff to assist him. What a thrill just to get outside and see something different. What a boost to the appetite to say nothing of the effect upon morale. It takes a little extra effort on the part of the staff, but pays tremendous dividends.

ACTIVITIES OF AMBULATORY PATIENTS

Ambulation is the process of moving from place to place in an upright position and includes bearing weight on the legs. For the disabled aged, it may differ slightly from what is thought of as normal walking. "Getting back on one's feet" is an age-old concept that symbolically marks the turning point in the road to recovery. Psychologically, the patient feels less confined if he is up on his own feet rather than chair-bound.

Ambulatory patients, even those with crutches or canes, can get into and out of areas too narrow to accommodate the wheelchair. Many times a patient will alternate ambulation with wheeling, depending on his needs and activities.

Before ambulation is planned for a patient, the entire rehabilitation team again evaluates the patient's abilities, limitations, and progress. After hearing each team member's report, the physician makes the final decision regarding ambulation.

A few patients, who have a minor disability, will be able to walk without any special assistance. However, when the patient first begins to ambulate, someone will need to provide support and a little help. Soon, however, the patient will become quite independent.

Other patients with more severe disabilities will require special aids to help them walk, such as artificial limbs, braces, canes, crutches, or walkers. Artificial limbs will be discussed in Chapter 8.

BRACES

Braces may extend the full length of the leg or go only to the knee. They have long metal rods that are attached to the patient's shoe and are used to stabilize weakened, paralyzed, or unsteady limbs. The physician orders the type of brace required, and the prescription is filled by an orthotist, a specialist in the construction and maintenance of braces and prostheses.

Health care personnel should know how to keep the brace in good repair. Metal joints should be oiled weekly with fine machine oil such as sewing machine oil. The appliance should be handled carefully to ensure the maintenance of proper alignment. Braces, like people, need an annual checkup. The patient is instructed to have the orthotist examine the brace yearly.

Nursing personnel will put the brace on until the patient has learned to do this for himself. Locomotion will be taught in the physical therapy department. When the brace is removed, the patient's skin should be inspected for any signs of pressure. If any redness is observed, the physician and the orthotist should be notified. The brace may need alterations or adjustments. Initially, the appliance should be worn only for short periods; then it should be worn for longer and longer periods of time until it can be worn all day.

WALKERS

Walkers are small metal stands that the patient leans on as he walks from place to place. They may be equipped with wheels and pushed around, or they may be moved by lifting. Some walkers have seats so that the patient can rest when necessary. Walkers are ordered by the physician and obtained from a surgical supply house. The technique of using the walker will be taught by the physical therapist.

CANES

Canes are sticks that the patient leans on to balance himself as he walks. Regular canes provide one point of support, have a curved handle, and are made of metal or wood. Broad-based canes have three or four prongs, which provide a wider base of support than the regular cane. Nonslip tips should always be applied to the end. The proper length for a cane can be determined by measuring from the patient's greater trochanter straight down to the floor. The greater trochanter is the large bony prominence on the hip and can be felt by slightly flexing and extending the patient's hip. Since canes provide only limited support to the ambulatory disabled, the patient must have a very slight handicap and be able to walk very well in order to use only a cane.

CRUTCHES

Crutches are walking-aids that are held in place by the arms. In fact much of the weight bearing is done by the arms, hands, and wrists. There are several kinds of crutches: underarm crutches (adjustable or nonadjustable), Canadian elbow extensor crutches, metal forearm crutches (also known as short Canadian crutches), and Kenny sticks. The physician will determine the type of crutch to be used and will so specify in his written orders.

Underarm crutches are held in place by the axillae, wrists, and hands. Weight is borne by the triceps muscles and not the underarms. In order to avoid any pressure on the axillary area, the crutches must be of the proper length. There are two main methods of measuring for underarm crutches. Nurses should realize that neither measuring technique guarantees the proper crutch length for every patient. When the patient begins to use the equipment, the crutches may have to be adjusted for greater ease and proper support. Thus, it is best to utilize only adjustable crutches, since they can be altered when necessary.

The patient should be standing when the crutch measurements are taken. Another person may have to support the patient while he stands. If it is impossible to have the patient in a standing position, he may be measured in bed, although this method is not as reliable as the standing method. Two measurements are needed: the total crutch length and the height of the handgrip.

The patient should wear his walking shoes when he is being measured. These should be Oxfords with good support, low rubber heels, a leather sole, steel shanks, and a firm counter. Good posture is essential if the measurements are to be accurate.

Standing Method of Measuring for Underarm Crutches

To obtain the crutch length, use the following procedure:

1. From the tip of the toe, measure 2 inches out to the side. Mark this point.
2. Measure 6 inches straight ahead from the first mark. Make a second mark at this point.
3. Measure from 2 inches below the axilla to the second mark. *This measurement is the crutch length.*

To measure for the handgrips, use the following procedure:

1. Have the patient make a fist with his wrist slightly hyperextended and flex his elbow to a thirty-degree angle. The handgrip will be placed so that it will fit into the fist.
2. Measure from the fist to the second mark on the floor to determine the placement of the handgrip on the crutches.

Bed Method of Measuring for Underarm Crutches

To obtain the crutch length:

1. Have the patient lie on a firm mattress and with good body alignment. Put on his walking shoes.
2. Measure 6 inches out from the bottom of the heel. Mark this point.
3. Measure 2 inches below the axilla to the mark on the bed. *This measurement is the crutch length.*

To adjust handgrip placement:

1. Obtain adjustable crutches.
2. Have the patient lie in bed with his shoes on.
3. Place the crutch 2 inches under the arm with the tip at the mark 6 inches from the base of the heel.
4. Have the patient make a fist, and flex his elbow to a thirty-degree angle.
5. Position the handgrip accordingly.

Usually underarm crutches are equipped with foam rubber axillary pads. Rubber suction tips are always placed on the ends of crutches in order to prevent slipping. These tips should be at least 2 inches in diameter. These additions to the basic crutch may extend the overall length of the crutch by ½ to 1 inch. Measurements must allow for the thickness of tips and pads.

Kenny Sticks and Metal Forearm Crutches

Kenny sticks and metal forearm crutches, or short Canadian crutches, are held in place by a cuff encircling the forearm and a handgrip. When measuring for this type of equipment, one must determine the handgrip height and the distance from the handgrip to the forearm cuff. The patient should stand in the same fashion that he would to have underarm crutches measured.

Standing Method of Measuring for Metal Forearm
Crutches and Kenny Sticks

To obtain the handgrip height:

1. Measure from the tip of the toe to 2 inches out to the side. Mark this point.

2. Measure 6 inches straight ahead from the first mark. Make a second mark at this point.
3. Have the patient make a fist with his wrist slightly hyperextended and flex his elbow to a thirty-degree angle.
4. Measure from the fist to the second mark on the floor. *This measurement is the height of the handgrip.*

To obtain the forearm cuff height:

1. Keep the patient in the same position.
2. Measure from the fist to 1 inch below the elbow. *This measurement is the height for the forearm cuff.*

Bed Method of Measuring for Metal Forearm Crutches and Kenny Sticks

To obtain the handgrip height:

1. Have patient lie on a firm mattress and with good body alignment. Put on his walking shoes.
2. Measure 6 inches out from the bottom of the heel. Mark this point.
3. Have the patient make a fist, with his wrist slightly hyperextended and flex his elbow to a thirty-degree angle.
4. Measure from the mark on the bed to the fist. *This measurement is the height of the handgrip.*

The measurement for the forearm cuff height will be taken in the same way as when the patient is standing. Again the measurement must allow for the use of a crutch tip.

OBTAINING THE EQUIPMENT

Crutches, walkers, and canes may be ordered from surgical supply houses. Many community agencies have loan closets that supply equipment on a temporary basis. Examples of such agencies are Elks clubs, Moose clubs, Kiwanis clubs, and some public health departments.

In some rural areas, where there are no sources for the purchase of this type of equipment, the nurse may have to rely on catalog mail orders. The purchasing agent for the local hospital or nursing home may have such catalogs available. Certainly, accurate measurements and adjustable equipment are essential for successful catalog purchasing. Any unacceptable equipment must be returned immediately. Mail ordering can cause a lengthy delay in the ambulatory process, and for this reason it might be wise to recruit a family member to make a trip to purchase necessary equipment. The buyer should be given the proper measurements, and the name and a picture of the article to be purchased. Furthermore, the measurements and other details should be recorded on the patient's chart. If the relative should lose the necessary information, he could call the nursing unit for the information.

PREPARATION FOR CRUTCH WALKING

Before the patient is taught to crutch walk, the doctor will prescribe special exercises to strengthen the muscles of the upper extremities that will be used for weight bearing. The patient will practice these under the supervision of the physical therapist. Nursing personnel should accompany the patient to the therapy unit and observe the exercises so that they can support the routine in the nursing care unit. Transfer procedures will be taught by the physical therapist, since details of the technique vary with the type of crutch. Walking or gait patterns will also be taught in physical therapy.

Nursing personnel need to know the basic gaits if they are to assist and encourage the patient in crutch walking as he performs the activities of daily living. The proper stance is essential for the patient to maintain proper balance and appearance when crutch walking. The patient should stand erect with his crutches 4 to 6 inches in front, and slightly to the side, of each foot. This stance will provide a good base of support. The weight should be on the palms of the hands with the wrists slightly extended and the elbows flexed at a thirty-degree angle. If the patient is using underarm crutches, these may press against the side of the chest to provide additional support. At *no time* should weight be borne on the axillary bar, since this could cause damage to the nerves in the axilla and subsequent loss of muscle function in the arm.

CRUTCH WALKING GAITS

A variety of gaits have been developed to meet the needs of patients with various lower limb weight-bearing problems. The doctor and the physical therapist decide on the gait pattern to be used by the patient. Most often the four-point or two-point method of crutch walking is the means of locomotion employed by the elderly.

The four-point alternate crutch gait is considered the safest and most stable of all the gait patterns. It is a good method for the elderly, who are frequently concerned about loss of balance. In order to use the four-point gait, the patient must be able to bear considerable weight on his lower limbs. This pattern is:
  1. Advance right crutch.
  2. Advance left leg.

3. Advance left crutch.
4. Advance right leg.

If the patient has a lower limb injury, he will be instructed to begin the gait pattern with his stronger leg. This is a slow method of locomotion, but it is usually ideal for the aged.

The two-point alternate gait is a faster method of walking, but the patient must have moderately good balance. This gait pattern resembles normal walking. The pattern is:

1. Advance right crutch and left leg.
2. Advance left crutch and right leg.

For both the three-point gait and the swinging gait, the patient must have considerably good balance and coordination. Generally, these gaits are used when weight can be borne on only one lower limb. The patient's arms must be very strong, since they will be supporting the weight of the entire body. These gaits provide a rapid means of locomotion, but because of the physical demands they place on the patient, they are generally contraindicated for the elderly.

As the patient becomes skillful in crutch walking, he should be encouraged to use this method of locomotion while performing activities of daily living. He should crutch walk to the bathroom, dining room, and therapy units. Health care personnel will need to arrange the environment so that the patient can ambulate with ease and still complete the ADL. Remember that both of the patient's hands are now occupied full time, and he cannot carry towels, soap, toothbrush, etc., to the bathroom. All necessary items for shaving, bathing, and oral hygiene must be at the location where these activities will be performed.

Nurses must observe the patient for signs of tiring and overexertion. Some patients think that once they know how to crutch walk, there is no reason for them to sit and rest. They consider having to use a wheelchair a personal insult. Common sense must be used when working with the elderly crutch walker. Perhaps the wheelchair would be advisable for long trips to therapy or diagnostic units. The patient needs to understand the reasons for not always crutch walking. Furthermore, he should know that wheeling is not considered a failure or a regression in his rehabilitation, but is an appropriate alternate at certain times.

PREPARING FOR DISCHARGE

Just as the process of rehabilitation begins at the onset of illness, so too, planning for the patient's discharge should begin early—as early as the day of hospital admission. Planning for discharge involves many people, and many factors are taken into consideration. The patient, rehabilitation team, patient's relatives or friends, and representatives of community resources all play vital roles. Perhaps the first consideration is where the patient will go following discharge from the rehabilitation unit—to another location within the same facility?—to a nursing home?—to a rooming or boarding house?—to his own home? the answers to these questions depend on: (1) the patient's physical and mental condition, (2) the willingness and ability of his family or friends to assist in patient care, (3) the availability of acceptable facilities in the community, and (4) the success of rehabilitation.

Perhaps the patient has no relatives living nearby, only a close friend. Can this friend assume responsibility as a substitute relative? What discharge plans will be made for the elderly who are totally alone? For the patient who will not be returning to his own home, the task of finding a suitable "home" is not an easy one. Sometimes it takes a considerable period of time to locate an acceptable facility that meets the needs of the patient as well as the family's financial limitations. Therefore, planning the discharge should begin early. Whenever feasible, the patient should be an active participant in selecting his next home. If the patient can visit the home under consideration, it might help him to make a sound decision. If this is not possible, the patient must be prepared in advance for discharge with explanations of where he will go and descriptions of his new home.

Once a tentative decision has been made, the nurse is in a unique position to help make the patient's adjustment to the new facility as smooth as possible. During the rehabilitative process the patient's progress has been recorded by all members of the team. This wealth of information should be shared with those workers who will be giving care after the patient leaves the rehabilitation unit. This is essential if the patient is to progress in rehabilitation or maintain his present level of functioning. If the unit to which the patient is being transferred is located within the same general facility as the rehabilitation unit, the staffs of the two units can share information at conferences. Or information may be relayed by means of written referrals from the rehabilitation staff to other agencies, such as a nursing home. The public health nurse who acts as coordinator may be instrumental in building a bridge between the rehabilitation institution and nursing home.

The information that is relayed must indicate in sufficient detail those activities of daily living that the patient can perform with and without assistance and include any pertinent information that will assist the new staff in caring for the patient and encouraging him to maintain previous accomplishments. An adequate and effective referral system provides the vital link in the chain of information connecting the known to the unknown.

If there is a possibility of the patient's returning to his own home or a relative's home, other factors need to be considered. The physical therapist may visit the home in order to determine whether or not the environment will need to be changed to accommodate the patient's disability. Can necessary changes be made with a minimum of cost to the family? For example, are the doors of the home sufficiently wide to allow for passage of the patient's wheelchair? Other health care workers may be asked to do home evaluations. The local public health or visiting nurse association may be called upon through written referrals from the physician.

Many aspects of the home need to be evaluated. Is the home under consideration the patient's private home? Is it one-story or two-storied? Is it an apartment—with or without an elevator? The problems facing the wheelchair patient living in a one-story single-family dwelling differ considerably from those of the wheelchair patient who has a home on the fourth floor of a walk-up apartment building. For those who plan to return to a rooming house or boarding house, the location and condition of the shared bathroom and kitchen can be serious barriers to a satisfactory adjustment.

The evaluator will consider the general layout of the home and note safety hazards that should be corrected if possible. Are there steps leading to the entrance? How steep are they? Are there railings to grasp while ascending or descending the steps? Can the family build a ramp so that the wheelchair patient can enter and leave the house with a minimum of effort? Can the patient using a wheelchair or walker maneuver about the house and through doors, or are doorsills an additional obstacle to locomotion? Throw rugs and highly polished floors are potentially lethal for everyone, but especially for the handicapped. The evaluator will need to discuss with the family the reasons for removing the environmental hazards.

The location of the bathroom and bedroom can be factors in deciding whether or not the facility is suitable for the elderly. If stairs must be climbed to get to the bedroom, the patient may find them an insurmountable barrier. Alternatives may need to be considered. Can the dining room be converted into a bedroom? If a bathroom is not nearby, can a commode be used in the bedroom? How will these changes affect the normal functioning of the family unit?

The bathroom evaluation will involve a consideration of the ease with which the patient will be able to effect transfer to and from the toilet, shower, and tub. Will grab bars, right-angle bars, elevated toilet seat, etc., need to be installed? The family will need to know what these are, where they can be obtained, how much they cost, and how they can be installed.

If the patient will have to do his own cooking, the kitchen will be visited. The height of kitchen surfaces in relation to the wheelchair or walker will be determined, and any necessary modifications will be indicated.

The full report will be submitted to the rehabilitation team for review. The evaluator will be asked to clarify certain points during the conference. As a result of the findings, the team may decide that weekend home visits will help the patient to make an easier adjustment to his home after leaving the rehabilitation center. These weekend visits provide the patient with a taste of what modifications he must make in self-care activities. It provides his family with a taste of what it will be like to have the patient home again. It allows both the patient and his family time to adjust gradually to this new situation.

The elderly disabled person may have to learn special activities prior to discharge. Outdoor locomotion may be a problem even though the patient may have mastered crutch walking in the physical therapy unit. Getting in and out of a car or bus, stepping off curbs, walking on uneven pavement, ascending and descending steps—all these may require new techniques to accommodate the patient's disability.

Once the patient has been discharged, active rehabilitation does not end. Visits from the public health nurse, physical therapist, speech therapist, and others may be ordered by the physician. These health team members report the patient's progress to the physician. Some patients may receive home care from the hospital following discharge—thus continuity of care is maintained. The wheelchair, braces, and other mechanical devices should be checked at intervals to assure their safe, effective functioning.

Although members of the health team continue to assist the patient in rehabilitation, it is the family or family substitute who now assumes the major role. The family now takes over the role of supporter and encourager as the patient achieves independence. There will be good days and bad ones for the patient, just as there were in the hospital. It is the loving family or friend who helps to make the transition period as easy as possible. It has been said that the real test of effective rehabilitation is the individual's ability to maintain his maximum level of functioning for the remainder of his life. A persevering patient, surrounded by love, and dedicated allied health workers form an unbeatable team in reaching this goal.

STUDY QUESTIONS AND PROBLEMS

1. When patients begin to take care of their own personal hygiene, it takes them a long time to accomplish simple tasks. This can be a frustrating experience for both the patient and the nurse. What can be done to alleviate this feeling of frustration?
2. List community resources where canes, crutches, and walkers can be purchased, rented, or borrowed.
3. The physical therapist has made a home evaluation visit and determined the need for equipping the bathroom with a raised toilet seat and right-angle bars. Where can these be purchased?
4. Most handicapped persons are unable to take advantage of social and recreational opportunities in the community, since public buildings are rarely designed to meet their needs. When new buildings, such as libraries, churches, and theaters, are being planned, what special features need to be included so that the handicapped can utilize the facilities?

BIBLIOGRAPHY

A Handbook of Rehabilitative Nursing Techniques in Hemiplegia. Minneapolis: Kenny Rehabilitation Institute, 1964.

Anderson, Helen C. *Newton's Geriatric Nursing.* 5th ed. Saint Louis: C. V. Mosby, 1971.

Ballantyne, Donna. "Evaluating ADL at the Bedside." *American Journal of Nursing,* November 1966, pp. 2440–2441.

Beland, Irene. *Clinical Nursing: Pathophysiological and Psychosocial Approaches.* 2nd ed. New York: Macmillan, 1970.

Carnevali, Doris, and Breuchner, Susan. "Immobilization: Reassessment of a Concept." *American Journal of Nursing,* July 1970, p. 1503.

Griffen, Winnie; Anderson, Sara J.; and Passos, Joyce. "Group Exercise for Patients with Limited Motion." *American Journal of Nursing,* September 1971, p. 1742.

Halley, Lydia. "The Physical Therapist—Who, What and How." *American Journal of Nursing,* July 1970, p. 1521.

Hirschberg, Gerald G.; Lewis, Leon; and Thomas, Dorothy. *Rehabilitation: A Manual for the Care of the Disabled and Elderly.* Philadelphia: J. B. Lippincott, 1964.

Homemaking Aids for the Disabled. Rev. ed. Rehabilitation Publication, no. 710. Minneapolis: American Rehabilitation Foundation, 1967.

Larson, Laura. "How to Select a Nursing Home." *American Journal of Nursing,* May 1969, p. 1034.

Lowman, Edward, and Klinger, Judith L. *Aids to Independent Living.* New York: McGraw-Hill, 1969.

Little, Dolores, and Carnevali, Doris. *Nursing Care Planning.* Philadelphia: J. B. Lippincott, 1969.

Martin, Nancy; King, Rosemarie; and Suchinski, Joyce. "The Nurse Therapist in a Rehabilitation Setting." *American Journal of Nursing,* August 1970, pp. 1694–1697.

Mitchell, Helen; Rynbergen, Henderika; Anderson, Linnea; and Dibble, Marjorie. *Cooper's Nutrition in Health and Disease.* 15th ed. Philadelphia: J. B. Lippincott, 1968.

Rossman, Isadore. *Clinical Geriatrics*. Philadelphia: J. B. Lippincott, 1968.

Roth, Julius A., and Eddy, Elizabeth M. *Rehabilitation for the Unwanted*. New York: Atherton Press, 1967.

Sorenson, Lois, and Ulrich, Patricia. *Ambulation: A Manual for Nurses*. Rehabilitation Publication, no. 707. Minneapolis: American Rehabilitation Foundation, 1966.

The Physical Therapy Manual for Physicians. Des Moines: Iowa State Department of Health, 1968.

West, Wilma. "Occupational Therapy Philosophy and Perspective." *American Journal of Nursing*, August 1968, p. 1708.

Restorative Nursing of Patients with Diseases of the Skeletomuscular System

ARTHRITIS

It is estimated that approximately 13 million Americans suffer from arthritis, the number one crippler of all age groups in the United States. It ranks second, after heart conditions, as the cause for limitation of activity in the older age population. Arthritis means inflammation of the joints and includes a number of specific diseases. The main types are osteoarthritis and rheumatoid arthritis.

Rheumatic disease of the joints does not respect age, sex, or race. Young children, as well as men and women, can suffer from rheumatoid arthritis. However, it most commonly occurs in women during the fourth and fifth decades of life. It is three times more common in women than in men and has been reported in 15 percent of the women over sixty-five. Nearly everyone over fifty is affected by osteoarthritis, causing 10 percent of this group to complain of pain.

Arthritis is one of the oldest chronic diseases known to man. Prehistoric bones from Egypt show evidence of the disease, and Hippocrates described a disorder that is almost the same as what we know as arthritis today. History records many famous people who have had arthritic disease—President James Madison, Mary, Queen of Scots, and the artist Pierre Renoir, to name a few.

The person afflicted with rheumatic disease should seek the help of a competent physician, preferably a rheumatologist, a doctor who specializes in the diagnosis and treatment of arthritis. The treatment is highly individualized, and the planning and care are usually done by a team, including both the physical and occupational therapists. Many arthritics become discouraged with the length of the treatment and their slow progress, and for this reason they may seek the services of those outside the medical profession—better known as quacks. These people prescribe all sorts of "cures" for arthritis, including magnetic charms, copper bracelets, special diets, prolonged fasts, large doses of tonics, mineral waters, herbs and seeds, and even large quantities of vinegar and oil. Many magazines and newspapers include advertisements for quick cures for arthritis and other chronic diseases. People will try anything when they are desperate and will reach out for whatever offers them hope. There is no quick and easy treatment for arthritis, and there is no cure. But people need not suffer from disabling symptoms. They can be treated.

RHEUMATOID ARTHRITIS

Rheumatoid arthritis is an inflammatory disease of the tissue lining the joints or the synovial tissue. This lining becomes swollen and thickened, and the synovium grows over the cartilage, destroying it and leaving bone and scar tissue in its place. In time and without treatment, the involved joint may become permanently stiffened (ankylosis). The joint capsule and ligaments may also become inflammed, stretched, and destroyed. These joint changes cause pain and muscle spasm. If these conditions are not corrected, deformities and flexion contractures will develop. Another problem that may occur is joint dislocation. The tendons may be affected by stretching and may rupture, causing the patient to lose use of the joint. Tendon changes occur especially around the hand and the wrist.

In an acute case of rheumatoid arthritis, the inflammatory process may affect the lungs in the form of pleurisy or pneumonia. The arteries, heart, and kidneys may be affected when the disease is rampant.

The patient usually complains of swelling, redness, heat, and pain in one or more joints. Frequently, the symptoms are symmetrical; that is, the same joints on both sides of the body may be involved. A classic symptom is early morning stiffness, known as gel phenomenon. Arthritis may "burn out" in one joint only to appear in another. This disease is characterized by remissions and exacerbations.

In the aged the disease is usually of long standing, and varying degrees of deformity and permanent damage can be seen. Perhaps the permanent disabilities of the aged arthritic are a result of the type of treatment that was available in previous years. Today, statistics show that with treatment severe crippling can be prevented in 70 percent of all cases. When rheumatoid arthritis develops in those over seventy or eighty, the onset is rapid and shows a generalized involvement of the body.

The cause of rheumatoid arthritis is unknown. For a long time many physicians believed that the disease was caused by an infection in the body. Because of this belief, doctors removed anything from the body that could be removed—tonsils, teeth, and gall bladders. Of course, this treatment was not effective. Attention was then turned to the bowel as a source of infection, and many arthritics had the cleanest colons in the world, due to repeated enemas and colonic irrigations.

The current theory links rheumatoid arthritis to an autoimmune reaction in which the body produces abnormal antibodies. These are directed against the body's own tissues instead of foreign material. Another theory holds that an infection may trigger the autoimmune reaction.

There are no specific tests for the diagnosis of rheumatoid arthritis. However, several laboratory examinations may aid in the diagnosis. These include blood counts and sedimentation rates. The latex fixation test for the rheumatoid factor—a complex protein found in the blood of patients with this disease—is positive in 90 percent of the patients with rheumatoid arthritis. X rays of joints and a biopsy of synovial tissue may also be performed.

TREATMENT

There is no magic formula for the treatment of rheumatoid arthritis. Each patient's therapy is designed to meet his own particular needs. Many patients can be treated on an outpatient basis. However, those with acute manifestations of the disease will require hospitalization. Not all arthritics will require active rehabilitation, but many will benefit from this approach. The physician's choice of treatment depends on the location and stage of the disease. The established methods of treatment for rheumatoid arthritis include emotional and physical rest, physical therapy, drug therapy, and corrective surgery.

Rest

In acute stages of this disease the patient will be admitted to a general hospital and placed on a program beginning with bed rest and progressing to active independence.

The outpatient who has a chronic form of arthritis will find that he tires easily and requires more rest than the average individual. Fatigue and stress are common, and many arthritics find that they are exhausted by the late afternoon. It is unwise for any arthritic, aged or very young, to attempt to do too much in one day. There is always tomorrow—the work will wait. Retired individuals do not have to maintain the pace of those who are employed, and they should plan periods of rest, especially in the afternoon, in order to avoid fatigue, which may exacerbate the disease.

Splints, braces, and casts may be used in early stages of arthritis. These are part of the rest program and are designed to reduce acute pain and provide increased functioning in the involved joint. Exercise will be prescribed when the acute inflammation subsides.

Physical Therapy

The physical therapy program will be highly individualized for each patient. Usually, the physician orders exercise and some type of heat therapy. Exercises may be isometric, passive, active assistive, or active in nature. The goal of such activity is for the patient to achieve the fullest possible range of motion for each joint. An intensive period of exercise is not advised for these patients, since it is extremely fatiguing and stressful. The exercises should be repeated five to ten times at several intervals throughout the day. A period of rest should follow each exercise session. The physical therapist will teach the nursing personnel the specific exercises for each patient. Some slight pain or a pulling feeling may be experienced when the exercise is started. This should subside after a few minutes of movement. Should discomfort persist, the exercise program should be stopped and the physician consulted. Therapeutic programs of exercise are not designed to be painful ordeals.

Some patients will be taught to do their exercises in their own homes. Once they have been taught the correct movements, it is up to them to carry out the therapy routine. Family members may take part if the patient requires assistance. Certainly, the family should remind the patient to do what he has learned and to perform the exercises regularly. The visiting nurse can assist both the patient and his family by acting as a liaison between them and the physical therapist.

Application of heat to inflamed joints will reduce pain, increase circulation to the part, and reduce swelling and stiffness. Many times heat therapy will be administered just prior to the exercise program so that the patient can take advantage of the benefits derived from the heat treatment. The relief provided by heat is temporary, but it is a valuable adjunct to the overall treatment. Heat must be applied with great care. A burn over an already diseased area will increase the patient's problems and prevent his active rehabilitation.

Warm soaks are the easiest method of applying heat. The affected part is submerged in a bowl, basin, or tub of water. A warm tub bath or shower is particularly effective in relieving early morning stiffness. Since the patient will have difficulty moving, especially into the tub, care must be taken to be sure he avoids falls.

Contrast baths are good methods of applying heat to hands and feet. The patient will need two basins or a double sink for soaking his hands and a bath thermometer. One vessel is filled with cold water at 65° F., and the other with hot water at 110° F. Hands or feet are placed in the hot water and then in the cold water. An alternating schedule of hot and cold is followed:

1. 10 minutes, hot soak
2. 1 minute, cold soak
3. 4 minutes, hot soak
4. 1 minute, cold soak
5. 4 minutes, hot soak
6. 1 minute, cold soak
7. 4 minutes, hot soak
8. 1 minute, cold soak
9. 4 minutes, hot soak

Plastic wastebaskets or buckets may be used for contrast baths for the feet. Both containers may be placed in the bathtub for ease in drawing the water and to avoid spills during the procedure.

Hot packs or hot wet towels may be applied to a large joint when soaking is not practical. These are changed frequently and applied for a period of 10 to 15 minutes. Chilling the patient should be avoided. Sometimes the physician may order the application of cold in the form of ice bags for 15 or 20 minutes two or three times a day. Deep heat, such as diathermy, ultrasound, and microwave, may be applied in the physical therapy department. There is little danger of skin burns from this type of heat treatment, which is always applied by a qualified person in the physical therapy department.

Paraffin wax baths are an effective method of applying heat to hands, knees, and ankles. The paraffin is melted in the top of a double boiler and heated to a temperature of 125° F. The hand is dipped into the melted wax. When the hand is removed, the joint will be covered with a film of hardened paraffin. The procedure is repeated until the limb is covered with a thick layer of wax. The joint is then wrapped in a waterproof covering and a towel so that the heat will be retained. After the heat has diminished, which takes about 30 minutes, the paraffin may be peeled off and returned to the pot for reuse. Paraffin may be applied to larger joints with a paintbrush. The danger of using paraffin wax is easily seen. Burns may occur if the wax is too hot. The danger of fire is ever present. Also, the double boiler may be dropped when it is removed from the stove, creating a mess to clean up and a hazardous area for walking.

Hot-water bottles and heating pads do not provide the benefits of moist heat. Although they do give comfort and warmth, the danger of burns is enough to discourage their use.

Drugs

Many drugs are used to reduce the pain and inflammation of rheumatoid arthritis. They are selected carefully, since most of them have many dangerous side effects. The nurse must be alert for any adverse reactions to drug therapy. A current pharmacology text is an essential reference at every nursing station, and those caring for the patient should know the cause, effects, and untoward reactions of all drugs the patient is receiving.

The most frequently used drug is aspirin—in large doses. This should be given after meals or with some kind of food, since many patients experience gastrointestinal distress when taking this drug. Enteric-coated aspirin may be ordered to avoid this problem. The major side effects from salicylate therapy are gastrointestinal bleeding, nausea, ringing in the ears, and hearing loss. Aspirin is thought to be a causative factor in the development of peptic ulcers. Other drugs that may be prescribed are gold salts, antimalarials, phenylbutazones (Butazolidin, Tandearil), and indomethacin (Indocin). However, they should be utilized with caution, since severe side effects, some of which are irreversible, may occur. Narcotics are not usually prescribed for arthritics because of the danger of addiction.

For many years ACTH, or adrenocorticotropic hormone, and cortisone were thought to be the miracle drugs in the treatment of rheumatoid arthritis. Experience has shown that although these drugs produce relief of pain, the disease process continues. In fact, the steroids may produce Cushing's syndrome and other problems, which can be even more serious than arthritis. However, when more conservative approaches have not been helpful to the patient, cortisone may be prescribed. In some cases steroids may be injected directly into the painful joint. This localized treatment may be effective in relieving pain, and thus reduce the need for systemic medication.

As with any chronic disease the patient requires close medical supervision. The type of drug and dosage will have to be adjusted as the patient's needs change. He should never self-medicate, change the drug therapy, or take any other drug without consulting his physician. It is advisable for the patient to carry a card in his wallet stating the drug he is taking and the amount and frequency of the dosage. If he should require emergency treatment, this information is vital to prevent complications.

Corrective Surgery

For many years surgical treatment of arthritis was considered a last resort. It was thought that surgery could not be performed on an inflamed joint because it would cause more injury and damage. Consequently, surgery was reserved for those joints in which the disease had burned out. Today, joint surgery is performed early in the course of the disease and is a major factor in the prevention of deformities. In addition, severe deformities can be corrected, and many patients experience relief from long-term discomfort and pain.

The elderly may be reluctant to undergo surgical treatment of arthritic joints, and sometimes the physician may not recommend this type of treatment. Most people, however, seem to respond very well to this approach, and the period of postoperative rehabilitation is relatively short.

There are three main types of surgery that may be performed on the arthritic joint: synovectomy, arthroplasty, and arthrodesis. The synovectomy is an excision of the diseased synovial tissue and is performed in order to prevent a return of the inflammatory process. To be effective, this surgery must be performed before the joint is damaged.

Arthroplasty is the surgical repair of a joint. This procedure may be done in conjunction with the synovectomy. Arthroplasty is a general term, and the operation may include one or more of a variety of techniques. The surgeon may remove the diseased head of one or more bones of the joint. This may be replaced by a prosthesis, as in total hip replacement, which is discussed later in this chapter. Other measures include resection or division of muscle and tendon fibers in order to restore use of certain joints. This approach is most often utilized to correct deformities of the fingers and wrists. The correction results in increased function.

Arthrodesis refers to the fusion of a joint. When, for example, there has been severe degeneration of a knee joint, arthrodesis may be the only approach that will reduce or relieve pain and permit walking. The patient will be left with a stiffened knee joint, which means that his deformity will be increased, but the joint will be more stable and therefore more functional. When both knees are involved, the surgery is restricted to only one, since fusion of both joints would severely handicap the patient and reduce his capabilities.

Surgical repair of various foot deformities, such as bunions and claw toes, may be indicated. The correction of these problems usually brings rapid relief from pain and improved walking and weight bearing.

The period of hospitalization following joint surgery is usually short. Nursing care is aimed at preventing the complications that may arise from enforced bed rest. Of particular importance is maintaining the range of motion in all of the joints, since the disease process may arise later in presently uninvolved areas. Specific exercises for the operative joints will be ordered by the surgeon. These will vary according to the extent and location of the surgery.

Arthritic surgical patients will view their operation with hope, for they anticipate a relief from pain, a correction of deformity, and an improvement of function. And in most cases the hoped-for results have been accomplished. The patient will need encouragement at every step of the recovery process. His interest and expectations can be used as a basis for enlisting his cooperation and assistance during the rehabilitation period.

Most patients go directly to their own homes upon discharge from the general hospital. Referrals to the visiting nurse and physical therapist are essential, since some therapy will be necessary on an outpatient basis. Programs of rest, exercise, and medication will be supervised and adjusted by the physician as necessary.

Special Considerations

Nursing the arthritic patient requires patience, kindness, and above all, understanding. Consider the problems of the patient who has to live with good days and bad days. In the morning he can barely muster the strength and ability to open his aspirin bottle, although in the evening he can do this without any difficulty. Frustrating, indeed—depressing, certainly. Perhaps the most common feeling of all arthritics is that of discouragement. With this goes the fear of crippling and complete invalidism with total dependence on others. The nurse should be aware of these feelings in her patient and realize why they occur. The patient should never be thought of as a hypochondriac or a faker.

Patients need to be encouraged to assume as many responsibilities as possible, but the nurse should be alert for signs of overtiring and fatigue. Activities of daily living should be scheduled for those times when the patient can function best, thus allowing him to gain a sense of accomplishment by performing these tasks.

Relief of pain is essential, and the patient must maintain his drug therapy and have it adjusted when necessary. Furthermore, attempting to do too much may cause an increase in discomfort. Patients have to learn their limits and not overstep these bounds.

Arthritic patients will be tempted to assume the position that affords them the greatest comfort. Usually their joints are flexed, very often with pillows under the knees. Since these postures will lead to flexion contractures, they must be avoided. During the daytime the patient should be changing his position frequently. At night, splints may be used to prevent abnormal joint positioning. Turning may be a difficult and painful procedure, as any type of transfer activity may be. It is best for the patient to perform movement himself, for he knows just how to get out of bed without increasing pain or placing undue pressure on an inflamed joint. This may be an agonizingly long procedure, but the nurse does better to offer the patient help and give it when necessary than to increase the discomfort.

Many diets have been proposed as miracle cures for arthritis. There is no such thing. The patient needs a well-balanced, nourishing diet. Anemia is a common finding with this disease, so iron supplements and iron-rich foods may be recommended. Weight control is essential, since diseased joints can hardly be expected to carry excess pounds. Patients with hand and wrist inflammation and deformities may have difficulties with the mechanics of eating. The occupational therapist will teach the patient to use various aids to accomplish this activity of daily living. The elderly homemaker will also need to learn new and easier ways to prepare foods, lift and move pots and pans, and continue with her household duties.

Special attachments may be added to crutches so that weight can be borne on the forearms rather than the hands and wrists. Special corrective shoes may also be needed.

OSTEOARTHRITIS

Osteoarthritis is often attributed to wear and tear on the joints. It is more common than rheumatoid arthritis and is considered to be less damaging. The onset of the disease usually occurs after the age of forty, and its victims are older persons.

A wearing down, or degeneration, of the joint cartilage occurs and eventually leads to exposure of the underlying bone. As a result the synovial tissue becomes inflamed, because of injury from the roughened bone ends. Pain, swelling, and stiffness then follow, usually beginning in the fingers and the weight-bearing joints of the spine, knees, and hips. Heberden's nodes may occur at the last joints of the fingers. These enlargements do not cause disability but are somewhat disfiguring. Osteoarthritis does not cause generalized systemic disease, but disability can occur when the disease is present in the knees, hips, and spine.

The cause of osteoarthritis is unknown, but there are two theories regarding its development. One holds that the disease is a result of the aging process. Normal wear and tear on the joints and chronic irritation from overweight, poor posture, and one's occupation are contributing factors. The other theory holds that hereditary, endocrine, or metabolic factors may cause the disease.

Osteoarthritis is diagnosed by x-ray examination of the involved joints. The treatment is basically the same as for rheumatoid arthritis. Surgical treatment has been effective in restoring function to the hips and the knees. Reducing wear and tear on the joints by correcting posture and reducing weight is most beneficial.

FRACTURES

The third leading cause of limited activity for the elderly is back and lower extremity impairments. Reduced reaction time, visual difficulties, poor balance, weakened muscles due to prior illness (strokes), and sometimes mental confusion contribute to the high incidence of falls in this age group. Even so-called minor falls often result in fractures. Some of the reasons for the increase in the incidence of fractures in the elderly, particularly women over sixty, were discussed in Chapter 4.

The most serious fracture in the aged is the broken hip, and the complications resulting from this injury are a major cause of death. Elimination of hazards in the environment could vastly reduce the high rate of falls, thereby reducing the occurrence of fractures. Throw rugs, slippery floors, rugs and steps in need of repair, stairs without handrails are a few of these hazards. Nurses who live in areas where winter brings icy steps and sidewalks have ample opportunities to care for the elderly with hip fractures. Bone metastasis due to cancer in another part of the body is also a cause of fractures.

The most common hip fractures are those of the neck of the femur and the trochanter. It has been estimated that 75 percent of all elderly persons with fractures of the upper femur have a preexisting osteoporosis. This condition occurs almost exclusively in women.

The patient's symptoms vary according to the location of the injury and the type of fracture (simple, compound, impacted, or comminuted). Symptoms such as pain, inability to move the injured part, and shortening of the extremity due to muscle spasm may also be accompanied by signs of shock. The circulatory system of the elderly may have real difficulties in accommodating itself to this sudden injury. First aid measures include emergency treatment for shock and immediate immobilization of the injured part prior to moving the patient to the hospital. Diagnosis is made by x-ray examination.

Treatment

At one time treatment for hip fractures involved long periods of immobility—perhaps four months or more in traction. Deaths resulted due to the body's inability to tolerate lengthy bed rest. Today, with improved surgical methods in the field of orthopedics, the period of immobility can be decreased, and therefore, the prognosis becomes more favorable. The goal of treatment is to have the patient ambulatory and functioning as well as he was before the injury. This should be accomplished in as short a time as possible. If this goal is to be achieved, the fracture must be reduced, and some immobilization must occur in order for the patient to regain and retain proper bone alignment. Rehabilitation techniques must be applied in order to restore proper functioning. The method of treatment depends on the type and location of the fracture and the physical and mental condition of the patient. The physician will determine how well the patient can tolerate the period of immobility. What are the chances of the development of thrombi, hypostatic pneumonia, or renal calculi? Preexisting physical conditions such as cardiovascular or urinary difficulties must be taken into consideration. If the patient was mentally confused prior to the present injury, will enforced bed rest further compound the problem? Careful medical and nursing management of the patient with a lower extremity fracture is of critical importance.

There are two principal methods of treating the hip fracture: internal fixation, which is more commonly called hip nailing, and replacing the head of the femur with a prosthetic device. Both are surgical procedures. The latter is the more involved technique. If the fracture is impacted (one fragment of bone is held together by another fragment), the physician may decide against surgery. As the bone heals, some amount of deformity will result, but not enough to warrant subjecting the patient to surgery. The remainder of the discussion on hip fractures will center on care of the patient requiring surgical treatment and the rehabilitation involved.

Once the decision has been made concerning the diagnosis and treatment, the patient and family need to know what the next steps will be and why. Many elderly patients become extremely apprehensive when they hear the diagnosis. The thought of a friend who had such an injury and never recovered flashes through their minds. Both patient and family will benefit from calm reassurance that if everyone works together (the family, patient, physician, and health care team), the patient may regain independence. Unfortunately, at times the nurse has so many duties to perform during the initial admission of the patient that the last priority becomes that of allaying the patient's fears. The overwhelming fear of helplessness is not neglected by an alert and empathic nursing staff.

Whether hip nailing or hip replacement is selected as the method of treatment, the patient is usually placed in traction as an initial step prior to surgery. Traction, or pull on a part of the body, accomplishes two main functions. It prevents the bone fragments from being displaced and relieves muscle spasms. Russell traction or Buck's extension may be used. The frame for Russell traction includes a trapeze, which makes it easier for the patient to raise himself from the bed at intervals. Nursing care personnel should carefully explain the amount of activity the patient may perform using the trapeze and the correct method of using this device. Many elderly patients have a tendency to assume a rigid position in bed. Fear of further injury or pain may be the reason for this lack of activity. The nurse needs to encourage and help these patients to move within the confines of the traction.

Nursing Care

Principles of nursing care for the patient in traction are the same as those for the patient confined to bed. Meticulous care in prevention of decubiti, contractures of unaffected joints, and foot drop of the unaffected foot cannot be overemphasized. Hypostatic pneumonia is a serious complication for immobilized hip fracture patients, accounting for about 50 per cent of their deaths. A most important part of the nursing care of these patients is the encouragement of deep breathing and proper coughing technique. Elevating the head of the bed will help effective coughing. The nurse should explain why these techniques are necessary and assure the patient that coughing will not affect the injury.

Because it is painful for the patient to use the bedpan, bowel and bladder problems may arise during the initial period of immobility. If the fracture pan is used and the head of the bed raised slightly, this will aid in avoiding some potential elimination problems. The elderly fear accidents while using the bedpan, especially when they are unable to sit up. Because of these fears, they sometimes have a tendency to hold back the normal urge to defecate. The nurse should be alert to this possibility, encourage the patient in the use of the fracture pan, and remove the pan immediately after its use. Adequate fluid intake will also help to reduce the incidence of urinary tract difficulties.

Usually the body's response to the injury causes some amount of abdominal distress. Gas-forming foods and those that are difficult to digest should be eliminated from the diet. Since constipation is common during this time, preventive measures must be initiated immediately.

The physician's orders will vary according to his personal preference and the condition of the patient. Anticoagulant therapy may be instituted, since there is a high incidence of clot formation during immobilization. The patient's tolerance for medications that relieve pain and evening sedation must be carefully observed. Nursing personnel will find that the patient who is confused during the daylight hours may become even more disoriented during the night. Sedatives may increase his confusion, and this should be promptly reported to the team leader to prevent further complications. Side rails should be on the bed at all times, and a night light in the room is reassuring to the patient. The nursing staff needs to assist the confused patient in orienting himself to time and place. A clock and calendar within the patient's sight will aid in establishing these concepts.

The goal for the patient is ambulation, and measures must be instituted as early as possible to prepare the way. Of course, range-of-motion exercises for unaffected joints are started, and a plan devised for strengthening those muscles that will bear most of the patient's weight when active rehabilitation begins. Circulation can become sluggish during the period of immobility, and a secondary advantage of exercise will be improved circulation.

The physical therapist will teach the patient the exercises to be performed in bed in traction. Exercises to strengthen the arms and the unaffected leg should be started. The proper use of the trapeze will also help to increase the strength of the patient's arm, shoulder, and neck muscles. Nursing care plans must include provision for assisting and encouraging the patient in performing those exercises taught by the physical therapy staff.

One of the most important principles in caring for the patient in traction is the constant maintenance of the proper amount of weight. Weights will be effective only if they are hanging free from the bed. Under no condition should they be removed without the written order of the physician. At times the patient may say, "If only the weights were off, I could use the bedpan more easily." The nurse should explain in easy-to-understand terms why the weights cannot be removed.

Nursing Care of Patients Recovering from Internal Fixation

Internal fixation is accomplished by surgically inserting a stainless steel or Vitallium (a nonelectrolytic metal) pin, screw, or plate, which holds both fragments of bone together in proper alignment. The fragments that are united by this device will heal around the inserted metal. The device remains in place for the rest of the patient's life, unless some problem occurs.

The physician may order the patient placed back in traction immediately after the operation for one or two days to relieve muscle spasms. Unless the reason for temporary traction is explained to the patient, he may feel that the surgery was a failure, and that the traction spells the beginning of complete and total helplessness. A simple explanation can do much in the way of encouragement.

If the patient is not placed in traction, the physician will designate which side the patient is to lie on. Outward rotation of the hip joint must be avoided, and the patient is reminded to assume a toe-in position of the affected limb while in bed. Postoperative nursing care principles are the same as for other surgical procedures. They include careful observation for signs of hemorrhage, encouraging deep breathing exercises, and checking voiding. Narcotics should be used cautiously, since the patient cannot tolerate depressed respirations. Activities of daily living are encouraged as a means of alleviating the patient's feeling of helplessness as well as an aid to improved circulatory-respiratory function.

Postoperative exercises may be ordered by the physician and carried out by the physical therapist as early as the first postoperative day. These exercises are aimed at strengthening the unaffected leg as well as the affected one. The health care team plays a supportive role in encouraging the patient to perform these exercises three to four times per day. As soon as possible the patient is ordered out of bed in a wheelchair. Sometimes weight bearing may be permitted on the unaffected leg. Although it is a happy day when the patient receives this good news, new fears and apprehension cloud his mind. Such concerns as "The pin won't hold" or "I know I'll fall again" may be verbalized or not. Unhurried, simple directions and the nursing staff's assistance in this important step will help allay the patient's fears.

One-legged stand-up exercises precede ambulation with a walker. The physical therapy staff, following the physician's directions, will teach these exercises as well as use of the walker or crutches. Heat treatments and massage may also be ordered as a means of increasing circulation to the injured leg. Ace bandages or antiembolic stockings may be indicated during ambulation as precautionary measures. (See Figure 8-1.)

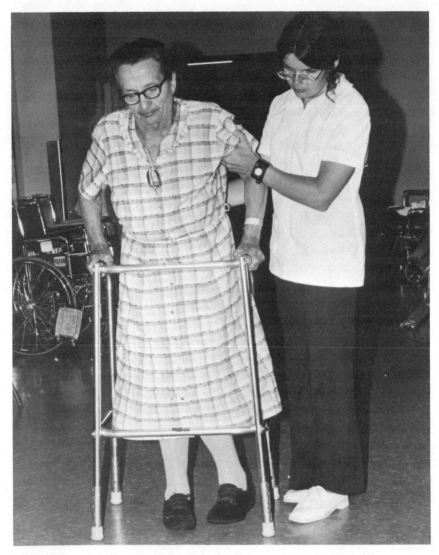

Figure 8-1: Ambulation with a walker following repair of a fractured hip.

The patient will be discharged before the physician orders weight bearing on the affected limb. The amount of weight bearing depends on the healing at the fracture site. A series of X rays during the period of convalescence records the healing progress. Trips to the physical therapy unit after discharge will be indicated. It may be three to eight months after hip nailing before full weight bearing on the affected limb can be accomplished.

Patients with a Hip Prosthesis

The physician may determine that the patient's condition and the type of fracture necessitate the removal of the fractured portion plus the neck of the femur. A metal prosthetic device is then inserted and anchored by means of a stem into the medullary canal of the bone. This is a complicated surgical procedure. Its advantage is the speed with which full weight bearing can occur and the relatively uncomplicated rehabilitation period. Following the surgery the patient may also be placed in traction for one or two days. Postoperative care is the same as previously discussed. Because there is a surgical wound, hemovacs (suction cups to drain the fluids from the area) will need to be carefully checked for bleeding and drainage. recorded. If there are no complications, the physician will order the patient out of bed with partial weight bearing as early as the second postoperative day. Independent ambulation is accomplished in about one month. At first, the walker will be used, then crutches, and finally a cane in order to support the weight on the affected limb.

Discharge

If there are no complications, the patient will be discharged from the general hospital unit within two weeks. The period of convalescence will take place at the patient's home, a nursing home, or a rehabilitation center. If the patient is returning home, the following items may need to be borrowed or purchased: a firm mattress or bed board, a walker, a wheelchair, and a commode. Arrangements will need to be made for the patient's return to the hospital or rehabilitation center for continued physical therapy treatments. The social service department of the hospital can help in seeing that transportation is available. In some instances home visits by the physical therapist may be required.

The patient and his family, with help from the nursing team, need to devise a daily schedule in which there is a balance of rest and activity. All concerned must realize that walking and doing other exercises to the point of fatigue can be dangerous and lead to another fall.

The doctor's specific orders must be reviewed so that the patient will understand what limitations are to be placed on his way of living. Usually, the continuation of a diet high in protein and calcium will help in the healing process. The family may need assistance from the dietitian in planning menus.

The patient will find it easier to get in and out of straight-back chairs, which provide firm support. Just as activities of daily living were encouraged by the staff during hospitalization, the patient needs continued support in performing these and other activities at home. Hazards in and around the home that could contribute to another fall must be eliminated. The aged person needs to understand why venturing out of doors when it is raining or ice and snow are present can be courting disaster.

Discouragement and depression may invade the elderly person who is recovering from a fractured hip. Early ambulation and short hospital stays may help to alleviate these feelings. However, the length of the convalescent period will naturally bring some depression. The family needs to understand that the patient will probably experience periods of frustration and irritability caused by the slow process of rehabilitation. This is particularly true of patients who have cherished independence throughout their lives. To be suddenly thrown into some form of dependence can be extremely difficult for the patient to accept. By working together, the family and rehabilitation team can help the patient to gradually regain his former independence and support him in coping with feelings of discouragement.

Some patients will not be able to return home directly from the hospital. For them the convalescent period will take place in a nursing home, an extended care facility, or a rehabilitation center. An adequate referral system should provide the information necessary for continuity of care.

AMPUTATION

Great strides have been made in recent years in rehabilitation techniques that assist the patient in making a satisfactory physical adjustment to amputation. Newer methods of manufacturing prosthetic devices and improved medical techniques have resulted from the treating of military casualties of World War II, Korea, and Vietnam.

It has been estimated that more than 75 percent of lower limb amputations are performed on those who are over sixty years of age. Two of the most frequent causes for surgical removal of a part or the entire limb are vascular disease due to arteriosclerosis and complications resulting from diabetes. Severe infection of the extremity and trauma may be additional reasons for amputation. The surgeon may amputate above or below the knee, depending on the circulatory conditions and other factors. The abbreviations AK and BK are used to describe the procedure. A below-the-knee amputation is more desirable, since the knee joint remains intact, and a satisfactory gait with prosthesis is accomplished more easily.

Preoperative nursing care includes heavy doses of psychological support for the patient. The surgeon will explain why the limb has to be removed. This explanation will also be given to the family members, so that hopefully they will be in a position to provide support during a most critical period in the patient's life. Caution must be exercised not to give reassurances that imply that total rehabilitation will be forthcoming. Unfortunately, not all elderly patients confronted with an amputation will progress to the point of total independence and full use of a permanent artificial limb. In many cases other physical conditions or disabilities render complete rehabilitation impossible. In some cases the patient's condition may be such that consideration of even a temporary prosthetic device is out of the question. Successful rehabilitation for this patient is accomplished when he is able to use the wheelchair effectively as the sole means of locomotion. The rehabilitation team should never consider this patient a failure. It is challenge enough to help him become a competent wheeler.

Preparing the patient for surgery includes other aspects in addition to psychological support and routine physical preoperative procedures. When feasible, the patient should be taught how to perform those exercises that will be used to strengthen his arm and leg muscles during the postoperative period. Also, preoperative practice in performing the transfer activities that he will use later (such as sliding boards) helps in postoperative adjustment. The physical therapy staff plays the major role in this aspect of preoperative care.

Each individual will react to the loss of a limb in his own way. The reaction will be determined by his experiences throughout life and will probably be similar to the way he has reacted to other stressful situations in the past. The patient may experience emotional suffering and grief over the loss prior to the actual amputation. The act of amputating the limb might be viewed as a severing of social ties with family and friends. Grief revolves around feelings of total helplessness, mutilation of the body, or social isolation. In this depressed state, the patient feels that life is no longer worth living. Sometimes he will refuse to acknowledge the loss —a defense mechanism known as denial. He will not look at the stump and will deny that it exists. The patient might benefit from talking with an elderly amputee who has made a successful adjustment and can share his experiences in a positive way. The nurse should be alert to the patient's concerns regarding his own body image and how he feels his family will react to him following surgery. Allowing the patient to verbalize his concerns may be more helpful than offering him trite reassurances.

The Patient Confined to Bed

General postoperative care for the elderly amputee incorporates the same principles of nursing care as for other surgical patients (encouraging the patient to move and cough, inspecting the dressings, observing for signs of bleeding, etc.). Attention must also be given to the prevention of complications, which would retard the patient's progress toward rehabilitation. Complications such as hypostatic pneumonia have already been discussed.

Individualized nursing care to meet the patient's physical and emotional needs is of prime importance. If, for example, the elderly amputee is also a diabetic the nurse must not only use her knowledge of basic postoperative care and of care for the amputee, but must also apply her knowledge of care for the diabetic patient. Adjustments in insulin and diet will have to be made for the diabetic amputee as he progresses in the rehabilitation program. Problems of the elderly diabetic will be discussed in Chapter 11.

Specific principles of postoperative care for the amputee include proper positioning of the stump to prevent flexion contractures of the hip and knee. The goal of postoperative care is to prepare the way for early ambulation and the effective use of a prosthesis by careful attention to the healing stump. The physician may order skin traction to the stump to aid in the healing process.

Bed exercises to strengthen the muscles of the patient's arms, shoulders, and trunk are also ordered in preparation for ambulation. The physical therapist will instruct the patient or reinforce instruction if the exercises were taught preoperatively. Range-of-motion exercises of the stump and unaffected limb will usually be ordered by the physician. Physical therapy treatments aimed at helping to increase circulation may be indicated. Placing the patient in a prone position without pillows under the hips will help prevent flexion contractures. The physician will indicate how frequently the patient should assume this position.

Some physicians prefer not to allow the elderly patient to get up out of bed until sufficient wound healing has occurred. The patient with vascular problems may, in the process of getting out of bed, injure the stump, causing the wound to break open. If the patient is allowed out of bed, he must be assisted by the nurse in such a way that trauma to the stump will be avoided.

When the amputation wound has healed, the stump will be prepared for a possible prosthesis. This involves shaping and strengthening the stump as well as controlling the amount of shrinking that the stump will undergo. Application of ace bandages to the stump helps in the shaping process. Careful attention to the skin underneath the bandages is a must, especially since circulatory problems are frequent among elderly amputees. The patient must be taught how to properly care for the stump as well as signs and symptoms of beginning infection or skin breakdown. The patient also needs to know that the stump will continue to shrink for about two years following surgery. (See Figure 8-2.)

The Patient Out of Bed

The physician will indicate when the patient is ready to begin ambulation. The plan for getting the patient out of bed will be based on his physical condition. Perhaps he will be too weakened for the one-legged transfer from bed to wheelchair or chair. Nevertheless, the nursing team uses those principles discussed previously in assisting with transfer activities. As the patient progresses in rehabilitation and his physical condition improves, the method of transfer will also be adjusted.

Once the patient is out of bed in a chair, exercise called chair push-ups may be ordered. In this exercise the arm muscles are used to lift the body off the seat of the chair, which prepares the upper extremity muscles for eventual crutch walking. Progress is then made to weight bearing on the unaffected limb. Practice on the parallel bars in the physical therapy department precedes instruction in the use of crutches and appropriate gait training.

Sometimes during the convalescent period the patient may complain of pain, numbness, or tingling sensations in the amputated limb. He may be reluctant to tell the nurse for fear of being ridiculed. This symptom is called phantom pain and is caused by nerves of the stump. These sensations usually disappear when the patient looks at the stump. Patients need reassurance that this is not an unusual symptom and that they are not going out of their minds. Most of all, they need psychological support in coping with this symptom.

Successful rehabilitation of the elderly amputee will depend on several factors. The general physical health of the patient must be considered. For example, the presence of vascular disease in the unaffected limb will vastly reduce the possibility of his participating in an active rehabilitation program. The diabetic amputee with accompanying visual difficulties is not a good candidate. Other problems may include osteoarthritis or osteoporosis.

The older the amputee, the slower he is to adapt to the prosthesis. For the patient aged seventy-five, the process of rehabilitation with prosthesis will probably be very slow. Of course, exceptions to the rule are

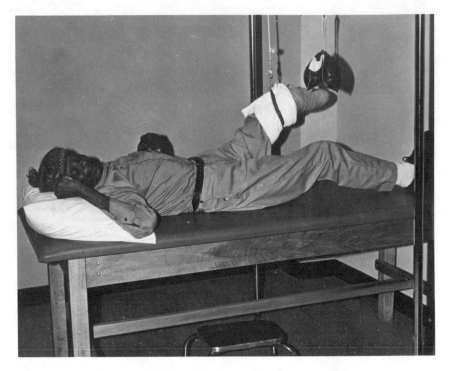

Figure 8-2: Exercising the limb in preparation for weight bearing on a prosthesis.

always a possibility. If the patient is determined to use the prosthesis and is highly motivated and challenged, rehabilitation can be accomplished in a relatively short period of time. Acceptance of the loss of the limb and insight into potential problems will help the patient during the period of rehabilitation.

When the patient has learned to crutch walk, the physician may discharge him before a permanent prosthesis is fitted, since the stump must be well shrunken and properly conditioned before a permanent artificial limb can be fitted. A temporary prosthesis, however, may be fitted to the stump before the patient's discharge, and it is usually well tolerated by the elderly amputee. The prosthetist will design and prepare the temporary device to assure proper fit. The physical therapy staff will then institute a program aimed at the patient's satisfactory adjustment and use of the device for locomotion. Teaching the patient to balance, place the prosthesis on the ground, and shift his weight from leg to stump and back—this is a part of the complicated rehabilitation process. Progress is made from parallel bars to crutches or canes, with the ultimate goal being total independence. Not all patients achieve this goal, however. The patient may become frustrated and revert to crutch walking without using the temporary artificial limb.

The technique of immediate postoperative application of a rigid dressing to which a temporary prosthesis is attached is becoming more widespread. A cast is applied to the stump while the patient is in the operating room. The purpose of the cast is to reduce the amount of edema and to help reduce pain. The lower end of the cast is designed to allow the attachment of a pylon, which is a tubular device that extends from the end of the cast to the floor and has an ankle and foot attachment. The advantage of an immediate postoperative artificial limb is the speed with which ambulation can take place. The patient can begin to bear weight as soon as the first day after surgery. This technique is particularly well adapted to the elderly amputee, because of his inability to tolerate immobilization.

Ambulation with the pylon begins with dangling and progresses to the patient's standing at the bedside and bearing slight weight on the affected leg with the support of a walker. The physician will gradually increase the frequency and length of time the patient spends standing at the bedside. The nurse reinforces the physician's instruction that the patient should not attempt to stand without supervision of the staff. The pylon must be attached when the patient is out of bed and removed when he is resting in bed in order to prevent skin breakdown.

The stump will, of course, begin to shrink during the healing process. The patient should understand that several changes of cast may be re-

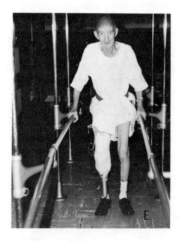

Figure 8-3: A typical patient 24 hours after a below the knee amputation. The stump has been fitted with a prosthesis during the surgical procedure.

quired, since early weight bearing seems to accelerate shrinking. The prosthetist will check the pylon for proper alignment each time the cast is changed, and required adjustments will be made.

The plan for ambulation, whether or not a pylon is used, will be individualized according to the physical and emotional tolerance of the amputee. The period of time it takes for the patient to progress from walker, parallel bars, crutches, and cane to total independence will vary greatly.

If the amputee handles the temporary prosthesis successfully, a permanent limb may be ordered. Another factor that needs to be taken into consideration is the cost. Prostheses are quite expensive. Will the patient derive enough benefit from the artificial limb to warrant such an outlay of money? Will the temporary limb serve the purpose? The physician and rehabilitation team members can help the patient to make a wise decision.

The patient will need to learn how to apply and remove the temporary or permanent prosthesis and the general care of the device. He has had to learn how to balance himself and ambulate safely. The more complex activities of daily living, such as walking up and down steps and ramps and managing curbs and uneven ground, take a long time to master. The patient will need the physical and emotional support of his rehabilitation family and of his own family and friends.

STUDY QUESTIONS AND PROBLEMS

1. Two weeks after the repair of her fractured hip Mrs. Benkle was discharged and went to the rehabilitation center. She had responded well to the hip nailing and had progressed to locomotion in the wheelchair. Her physician has requested that the rehabilitation team assist her in learning transfer activities and ambulation with support (walker, cane, crutches, etc.).

Mrs. Benkle will be seventy-nine in two weeks and is looking forward to a visit from her four children and ten grandchildren on that day. She is a widow who has her own room at her eldest daughter's home. Mrs. Benkle enjoys gardening, bingo, pinochle, and daytime television soap operas. The nursing staff agree that she is the most pleasant and cooperative patient in the rehabilitation unit.

The nursing staff has identified several nursing care problems that will be discussed during the team conference. What are some approaches that may be used in solving these problems?

a. Mrs. Benkle is afraid of falling and sustaining another fracture. Her fear is so great that she becomes stiff and rigid during the transfer procedure and consequently cannot use the toilet or the walker.

b. The patient has a tendency toward constipation and nighttime urinary incontinence. The latter is very embarrassing and humiliating to her, and therefore she prefers to sit in a wet bed instead of "bothering the nurse."

c. Mrs. Benkle's dentures and eyeglasses were broken when she fell. Her family has not been able to have these repaired, since she is unable to go to the dentist or optician.

d. Plants of every type and variety are on every surface in the patient's room. It seems that everyone who knows her has sent a get-well plant, and the room looks like a greenhouse.

2. Mrs. Leary, age seventy, has been transferred to a nursing home following a cholecystectomy. In addition to her surgery Mrs. Leary has been an arthritic for almost twenty years. During most of this period she did not seek medical relief for her arthritic symptoms, but relied chiefly on home remedies, including red flannel and her precious copper bracelet. The physician's goal is to help Mrs. Leary regain her strength while in the nursing home. Furthermore, she is to begin and learn range-of-motion exercises.

The nursing staff is angry with Mrs. Leary because she places more confidence in her copper bracelet than she does in her medical treatment. Discuss the attitude of the staff in this situation.

At the nursing care conference the staff members cite some problems in caring for Mrs. Leary. What can the nurse do to solve some of these problems?

a. Mrs. Leary experiences nausea from the large doses of salicylates she is receiving for joint inflammation and pain.

b. The patient is on a low-fat diet. She despises skim milk and loves bacon, ham, cream, eggs, etc. She is not overweight but is on a postoperative low-fat diet for a few weeks only.

c. She is unable to perform any ADL in the morning due to the gel phenomenon of rheumatoid arthritis.

d. She has been taught range-of-motion exercises in physical therapy and refuses to do them in the patient care unit. Mrs. Leary says that they are a meaningless, useless, and boring activity.

BIBLIOGRAPHY

Anderson, Helen C. *Newton's Geriatric Nursing.* 5th ed. Saint Louis: C. V. Mosby, 1971.

Beeson, Paul, and McDermott, Walsh, eds. *Textbook of Medicine.* 12th ed. Philadelphia: W. B. Saunders, 1967.

Bosanko, Lydia. "Immediate Postoperative Prothesis." *American Journal of Nursing,* February 1971.

Corrigan, Alfred. *Living with Arthritis.* Sidney, Australia: K. G. Murray, 1969.

Eyre, Mary. "Total Hip Replacement." *American Journal of Nursing,* July 1971.

Facts About Osteoporosis. Bethesda, Md.: National Institute of Arthritis and Metabolic Diseases, 1970.

Hirschberg, Gerald G.; Lewis, Leon; and Thomas, Dorothy. *Rehabilitation: A Manual for the Care of the Disabled and Elderly.* Philadelphia: J. B. Lippincott, 1964.

Homburger, Freddy, and Bonner, Charles. *Medical Care and Rehabilitation of the Aged and Chronically Ill.* 2nd ed. Boston: Little, Brown, 1964.

Larson, Carroll, and Gould, Marjorie. *Calderwood's Orthopedic Nursing*. 6th ed. Saint Louis: C. V. Mosby, 1965.

MacGinniss, Oscia. "Rheumatoid Arthritis—My Tutor." *American Journal of Nursing,* August 1968.

Marmor, Leonard; Walike, Barbara; and Upshaw, Mary Jane. "Rheumatoid Arthritis—Surgical Intervention." *American Journal of Nursing,* July 1967.

Myers, Julian S. *An Orientation to Chronic Disease and Disability.* New York: Macmillan, 1966.

Rossman, Isadore. *Clinical Geriatrics.* Philadelphia: J. B. Lippincott, 1968.

Schoenberg, Bernard; Carr, Arthur C.; Peretz, David; and Kutscher, Austin H., eds. *Loss and Grief: Psychological Management in Medical Practice.* New York: Columbia University Press, 1970.

Smith, Dorothy; Germain, Carol; and Gips, Claudia. *Care of the Adult Patient.* 3rd ed. Philadelphia: J. B. Lippincott, 1971.

U.S., Department of Health, Education, and Welfare, *Arthritis—Washington Health Report.* Washington, D.C.: U.S. Government Printing Office, 1968.

U.S., Department of Health, Education, and Welfare, *Arthritis and Research.* Washington, D.C.: U.S. Government Printing Office, 1968.

U.S., Department of Health, Education, and Welfare, *Arthritis and Rheumatism.* Washington, D.C.: U.S. Government Printing Office, 1967.

U.S., Department of Health, Education, and Welfare, *Diet and Arthritis.* Washington, D.C.: U.S. Government Printing Office, 1969.

U.S., Department of Health, Education, and Welfare, *Health in the Later years of Life.* Washington, D.C.: U.S. Government Printing Office, 1971.

U.S., Department of Health, Education, and Welfare, *Working with Older People—A Guide to Practice,* vol. 4, *Clinical Aspects of Aging,* Austin B. Chinn, ed. Washington, D.C.: U.S. Government Printing Office, 1971.

Walike, Barbara C.; Marmor, Leonard; and Upshaw, Mary Jane. "Rheumatoid Arthritis." *American Journal of Nursing,* July 1967.

Walike, Barbara C. 'Rheumatoid Arthritis—Personality Factors." *American Journal of Nursing,* July 1967.

9

Restorative Nursing of Patients with Diseases of the Nervous System and Special Senses

PARKINSON'S DISEASE

In 1817 James Parkinson first described the major symptoms associated with the disease that later bore his name. This slow, chronic, progressive disease of the central nervous system causes varying amounts of disability for approximately 1.5 million persons in the United States. It is estimated that about 50,000 new cases of Parkinson's disease are diagnosed each year. There is a higher incidence among men than women, and it affects the white race more than nonwhites. It does not respect geographical areas and can be found in all parts of the world.

The onset of the disease is usually between the ages of fifty and sixty, and it affects the motor nerves. The specific cause is unknown. Some researchers have indicated that a degenerative process may be a factor, but no conclusive evidence has been found.

Parkinson-like symptoms may also be found in patients with generalized arteriosclerosis, cerebral vascular lesions, or carbon monoxide poisoning and in those in the advanced stages of syphilis. For up to ten years after the encephalitis epidemic between 1919 and 1926, large numbers of persons displayed symptoms of Parkinsonism as an aftermath of encephalitis. Patients displaying Parkinson-like symptoms are said to have secondary or symptomatic Parkinsonism. This discussion, however, will center on patients displaying classic symptoms of Parkinson's disease, or paralysis agitans.

The basic symptoms of Parkinson's disease include akinesia (muscle rigidity), tremors, problems of the autonomic nervous system, shuffling gait, and masklike facies. Initially, only one side of the body may be affected. However, the disease progresses to bilateral involvement. The patient experiences a loss of dexterity and has difficulty arising from a bed or chair or initiating locomotion. He will make several attempts to change his position before he can accomplish this task. The muscles are rigid, and when the joints are moved by another person, a cogwheel effect can be felt in the muscles. There appears to be a deliberate slowness of motion, as if the patient were thinking out every action before performing it. He does, in fact, have great difficulty in controlling muscular activity and has lost normal spontaneous movements, such as freely swinging his arms while walking. The gait is a series of rapid, tiny, shuffling steps with the patient leaning forward. He seems to move his body as one solid unit, *en bloc*, rather than gliding along by shifting weight from one limb to the other. His posture is stooped with his head down and his elbows and knees slightly bent.

The tremor of Parkinson's disease is rhythmical and constant, occurring about five or six times a minute. These movements increase when the patient is walking or resting. The tremor of his hands and fingers has been described as pillrolling in nature. Even his tongue is affected by these tremors.

Other problems of the autonomic nervous system include increased salivation and lacrimation, constipation, urinary incontinence, and decreased sexual functioning. Speech is severely altered. It is slowed and almost monotonous in quality. The patient will notice a change in his handwriting. His signature becomes so radically altered that the bank may request a new signature card. The writing becomes tiny and decreases in size as the patient writes. This manifestation is called micrographia.

As the symptoms progress, the patient becomes withdrawn—almost a recluse. He can barely feed himself, swallow, or clothe himself, and has severe difficulties with recreational activities, such as shuffling cards or holding and placing bingo markers. The elderly Parkinsonian patient may become disoriented, aggressive, suspicious, and depressed. Hallucinations may also be present.

There are no specific diagnostic tests for Parkinson's disease. The neurological examination and the patient's manifestation of the basic symptoms of akinesis, rigidity, and tremor are sufficient to determine the diagnosis.

Treatment

Surgical treatment of this disease has not been successful with the elderly patient, and drug therapy is usually the treatment of choice. There is no cure for Parkinsonism, and the treatment is palliative.

A number of synthetic drugs are used to treat Parkinson's disease. They are called anticholinergics. Unfortunately, the side effects of these medications are most severe in elderly patients. The more effective these drugs are in controlling the symptoms of the disease, the greater is the likelihood of side effects. Urinary retention and mental symptoms, such as confusion and hallucinations, are possible side effects. Examples of these drugs are Artane, Disipal, and Cogentin.

The physician will prescribe small doses of the drug of choice and gradually increase the amount the patient is to take. This process is highly individualized. Use of anticholinergics is contraindicated when glaucoma, urinary retention, or tachycardia with heart disease is present. Sudden withdrawal of these drugs will produce Parkinson's crisis—an aggravation of the symptoms, causing the patient to become helpless and bedfast with severe mental confusion.

The most recent contribution to drug therapy has been L-dopa. This synthetic drug may reverse or reduce many of the disabilities caused by Parkinsonism. The rigidity and muscular problems diminish, and later speech improves and the tremors subside. The classic Parkinson's facies remain, however. Numerous side effects result from L-dopa, and these occur as the medication is increased to the patient's maximum tolerated dose. Some side effects are nausea, postural hypotension, and involuntary movements.

The adverse reactions to L-dopa are treated in a variety of ways. Nausea, for instance, may be relieved if the patient takes the medication with meals. Other drugs such as antacids or antiemetics may be prescribed by the physician. Often the symptoms will subside if the dosage of L-dopa is reduced.

As with the other anti-Parkinson drugs, the dosage of L-dopa is highly individualized for each patient. Small quantities are prescribed initially and increased until the physician has determined the optimum daily maintenance dose. Because there are many adverse physical and psychological reactions to this drug, the doctor will carefully and continually evaluate his patient.

Pyridoxine (vitamin B_6) has caused reversal of the therapeutic effects of L-dopa. Therefore, the patient should not take any multivitamins or vitamin supplements that contain this substance. The physician may request the patient to avoid foods that are high in vitamin B_6 content. Examples of these foods are powdered skim milk, legumes, sweet potatoes, yams, avocado, wheat germ, oatmeal, pork, bacon, tuna fish, beef, liver, and kidney. Other sources of pyridoxine are given in recent nutrition texts. Dried fruits, such as prunes, figs, and apricots, contain moderate amounts of vitamin B_6. Many patients utilize these fruits to help correct constipation. Dried fruits should be consumed in moderation, and other measures, such as adequate fluid intake, should be used to solve constipation problems.

L-dopa has been in use for only a few years, and research on it continues. The drug is not curative. Nor is it known that it alters the course of the disease. It has been reported that approximately 65 percent of Parkinsonian patients show some clinical evidence of improvement while taking this drug. However, almost all patients experience some side effects. The long-term effects of L-dopa on the patient and the disease process have not been established.

Nursing Considerations

Rehabilitation is centered on three main goals—reducing the amount of muscle rigidity, helping the patient to maintain a functional range of motion, and helping him to maintain functional use of his upper and lower extremities. If active rehabilitation is neglected at the onset of the disease, contractures and resulting deformities will occur, which vastly reduce the possibility of the patient's performing self-care activities and locomotion. Nursing personnel play an important role in assisting other members of the team—the physical therapist, occupational and recreational therapist, and speech therapist—in carrying out the rehabilitation.

The symptoms of Parkinson's disease are aggravated by stress and anxiety. The process of being admitted to a health care facility is an anxiety-producing experience for everyone and especially for this patient. Careful explanation of the institution's routines, orientation to the patient's immediate surroundings, and introduction to the various personnel and patients in the unit are most important in helping the patient to adjust to a strange new world. Although the patient's speech is impaired, his thinking process is not. The patient may be very alert and crave intellectual stimulation, even though his outward appearance shows a blank, emotionless expression. One-sided conversations with the patient can be emotionally taxing on the nurse, but they can provide that psychological boost to the patient's morale that is as important as caring for his physical needs.

The patient longs for emotional acceptance on the part of his family, friends, and members of the rehabilitation team. Nursing personnel must keep this fact in mind when caring for the patient or assisting him in caring for himself. A touch of the hand, a reassuring smile, and other nonverbal communications may convey acceptance without a word being spoken. When verbal communication is indicated, speak slowly and distinctly. Abrupt and hurried speech can produce stress for the patient, who can ill afford such an encounter.

Because of increased muscular activity, due to tremors and muscle rigidity, the patient will have an intolerance to heat. Room temperature should be adjusted to accommodate for this situation, and the patient's clothing should be light in weight.

Proper balance of rest and exercise is essential for the patient with Parkinson's disease. The physician will indicate how frequently exercises are to be performed, and a program will be devised in cooperation with the physical therapist. The nursing personnel should encourage the patient to perform the exercises that have been ordered. The nurse must be alert to signs of fatigue, so that alterations in the exercise program can be made. When the patient is fatigued, his symptoms tend to be exaggerated, and this can be most disturbing and discouraging to him.

The patient is encouraged to get out of doors once a day if possible, and the exercise program may include outdoor activity such as walking. It is up to the nursing personnel to reinforce directions given in the physical therapy department regarding walking technique. Some of the instructions that may need to be repeated in the patient care unit are: Touch the floor with the heel first; keep knees straight and body erect; lift foot to avoid scraping of the toe part of the shoe; and maintain a wide base of support. Some physical therapists teach the patient to clasp his hands behind his back when walking rather than to allow his arms to fall stiffly at the side. Whatever the directions, the nurse must know what the patient has been taught so that confusion can be eliminated and uniformity assured.

The major portion of the patient's day should be spent out of bed. However, rest periods in bed during the day are indicated. Bed boards and a firm mattress will provide adequate support. Because of the patient's tendency to bend forward, he should not use a pillow and should rest in the prone position as much as possible. Although insomnia is a problem for the patient, adequate amounts of exercise during the day can help reduce this annoying problem.

Although there is no cure for this disease, its progress may be reduced slightly if the patient is well nourished. Providing adequate nutrition presents many problems, however, for the patient, his family, and the nursing care team. The diet ordered will depend on the general physical state of the patient, the symptoms present and their severity, and the types of medications being given. The patient at home should eat with other family members as much as possible. This provides the social contact so necessary for the patient. Foods that are unlikely to spill should be selected whenever possible. Trying to get peas onto a spoon and up to the mouth can be terribly frustrating when arm tremors are present. Foods that are effective in combating constipation such as whole grain cereals should be included in the diet as tolerated. Inactivity and certain drugs contribute to the constipation problem. As the disease advances, drooling becomes a problem, and social dining at restaurants, etc., becomes restricted. This is most unfortunate, since the patient psychologically needs social outlets. He should be encouraged to feed himself as long as possible. In the later stages of the disease the patient will no longer be able to perform this function. Many patients become undernourished and dehydrated because of the difficulty they have swallowing and chewing. Another danger during the later stages is choking while attempting to swallow; such choking can lead to aspiration pneumonia.

Helping the patient to maintain independence in the areas of personal hygiene and other activities of daily living is an important aspect of nursing care. Learning to cope with muscle rigidity and tremors of the fingers, arms, and eventually the entire body is a slow process for the patient. The occupational therapist will teach the patient how to manipulate buttons, zippers, and snaps, which are essentials in his learning how to dress, and the nurse in the patient care area can encourage additional practice of these fine finger movements. Clothes that are easy to manage should be selected.

There will be periods when the patient will be frustrated by his inability to perform "simple" tasks such as buttoning his own shirt. Because of the emotional instability caused by the disease, the patient may vent his frustration by crying. This may cause further depression, particularly in men, since our culture unfortunately frowns on this kind of emotional release in males. Nursing personnel must show the patient that his behavior is acceptable, that she understands his frustration, and help him pick up the pieces and try again.

The family will also need to understand that psychological factors play a major role in the patient's ability to overcome his disability. The rehabilitation team works with both the patient and his family in providing psychological support. At home family members must encourage the patient, and if necessary, assist him in performing activities of daily living. Watching a loved one struggle to put on a shirt can be almost more than one can bear. Nevertheless, the family members must understand that they should not interfere and realize the psychological damage that would occur if they took over. Massive doses of encouragement, reassurance, and sympathy must be given to both the patient and the family in order to give them the psychological support necessary for them to tackle mounting difficulties as the disease progresses.

One of the patient's difficulties is lack of intellectual stimulation. As previously stated, the patient's level of intelligence does not diminish, even though his outward appearance may give that impression. Boredom creeps into the patient's life, and watching television does not solve the problem. When the therapist or nurse institutes recreational therapy, the patient's interests and ability must be considered, so that the diversional aspect of the activity is maintained. Busy work disguised as recreational therapy is useless and contributes to more boredom. Patients who like to write letters and find that their penmanship is not readable may learn to typewrite, which not only provides recreational and occupational therapy, but also provides the necessary exercise for the fingers. Recreation should also include group activities, since social isolation becomes an increasingly difficult problem as the disease progresses.

The speech therapist will plan a program aimed at assisting the patient in maintaining control of tongue and facial muscles, so that slurred speech can be corrected. The nursing personnel should encourage the patient to perform the exercises he has learned from the therapist. Some health care agencies have group exercise clubs, which are open to patients with Parkinson's disease upon referral from their physician. Inpatient and outpatient groups come together to practice speech control and to exercise in order to maintain their existing range of joint motion. The value of group participation is that of group support. It is comforting for the patient to know that he is not alone—that others have similar problems.

The nurse should be constantly alert to evidence of side effects caused by anti-Parkinson drugs. Blurred vision and confusion, two possible side effects, compound the patient's problem of locomotion. The aged are also prone to such side effects as dry mouth, constipation, and hallucinations. Prompt reporting of these symptoms is essential if further difficulties are to be avoided. Watching for symptoms of drug intolerance is an important function of the nursing staff. The patient and his family should also be taught these symptoms. However, they should be warned that the dosage of the drug should *not* be altered according to the way the patient feels from day to day. Other drugs, such as patent medicines, should not be used without the doctor's consent, since they may interfere with the anti-Parkinson drugs. Using drugs without the doctor's consent is like playing with dynamite!

As the disease progresses, the patient becomes more and more dependent on others. The family needs to be taught how to perform range-of-motion exercises and other techniques in caring for the patient. Families are encouraged to care for the patient at home as long as possible. Supportive help from the public health nursing agency or local homemaker service may be needed, and the necessary referrals should be made. When the family is no longer able to cope with the disease process, the patient is usually admitted to a nursing home, where he receives custodial care. The patient is highly susceptible to respiratory disease, and death usually results from pneumonia. The course of the disease runs about twenty years.

Although there is no known cure, research in recent years has produced drugs that help to control some of the disturbing symptoms. From time to time news articles appear that imply there are miracle cures for the disease. These provide vain hope for the patient and his family. With technical advances in the medical field, however, the day may come when the cause of Parkinson's disease is determined. Until that time nursing care and rehabilitation techniques will revolve around helping the patient to lead as normal and productive a life as possible.

CATARACTS

According to the National Society for the Prevention of Blindness, there are approximately 250,000 legally blind persons in the United States who are over sixty-five years of age. The two most common geriatric eye problems are cataracts and glaucoma.

A cataract is an opaqueness of the crystalline lens of the eye. Cataracts may be congenital, or present at birth, or they may develop during the middle years. Usually, however, they are found in the older adult. When cataracts occur in this age group, they are called senile cataracts.

Although there are many theories, the cause of senile cataracts is unknown. The symptoms produced by cataract development involve changes in vision. The patient will complain that glare and bright lights bother him and that his vision is distorted. He can no longer read or view television, and women are unable to do close handiwork such as crocheting, knitting, or embroidery.

The condition is diagnosed through eye examination by the ophthalmologist, and the treatment is surgical removal. There are several surgical techniques used to remove the lens and/or the capsule. The surgery is performed under local anesthesia.

When the patient is admitted to the general hospital, he should be psychologically prepared for the surgery. He needs to know that one or both eyes will be bandaged postoperatively (although only one cataract will be removed at a time and usually only the involved eye is bandaged).

Nursing personnel should orient the patient to his new environment and explain the daily routine of the hospital. Furthermore, the patient should know that side rails will be on his bed and why they will be there. Postoperatively the patient will be confined to bed for three or four days, and during this period his movements will be restricted in order to prevent tension on the suture line. The nurse should explain to the patient that his movements will be restricted in order to prevent postoperative complications. Nursing measures to promote comfort and prevent complications should also be employed.

The patient will have vision problems while using one eye, which may or may not be diseased. He will need assistance with activities of daily living until he can assume the responsibility for these tasks himself. Exercise will be limited for several weeks following surgery. Lifting, stooping, and bending must be avoided. The patient should walk with someone until he becomes accustomed to seeing with one eye.

If at any time during the postoperative period the patient is completely sightless, the nurse should always announce her entry into the patient's unit and explain all her activities. Careful planning of all activities of daily living is essential for the sightless patient.

The patient will be discharged with a dressing and a patch over the operative eye. The physician may prescribe temporary glasses after a few weeks. These provide fairly clear central vision, but because of the thickness and convex shape of the glasses, the patient's side vision will be distorted. The patient will have to turn his head for good vision, and his depth perception will be altered. He will need practice climbing steps and stepping onto curbs. Objects will appear about one-third larger than they are in reality. Contact lenses help to reduce the size of objects viewed and are frequently prescribed for unilateral cataract surgery.

Contact lenses are very small plastic lenses that are worn directly over the cornea of the eye. The lenses float on the fluid of the eye and are held in place by the tears and the upper lid.

The patient will be taught to insert and remove the lens by the ophthalmologist or contact lens technician. Some basic principles taught to those who wear contact lenses are:

1. Wash hands with soap and water before removing or inserting the lenses.
2. Clean the lenses with the proper cleaning solution and dry them before placing them in the storage container.
3. Keep storage container clean.
4. Remove the lenses if they are uncomfortable.
5. Do not wear the lens while sleeping or if the eye is irritated or infected.
6. Wear lenses only for the recommended time period.

Many elderly patients have difficulty removing the lenses and sometimes fall asleep with them in place. Sleeping with the lenses in place may cause injury to the delicate tissue of the cornea. Nursing personnel may have to assist the patient in removing his contact lenses. The patient should sit at a table and look straight down. He then extends the outer canthus of the eye with the middle finger of the hand. If the lens is in the right eye, he will use his right hand. The opposite hand is cupped beneath the eye to catch the lens. When the outer canthus is extended, the patient gently closes his eye. The pressure of the eyelids upon the edges of the contact lens will cause it to pop out of the eye.

Contact lens wearers should carry wallet cards stating this fact. In the event of a medical emergency, accident ward personnel would have to remove the lens with a special suction instrument.

Generally, most cataract patients have permanent corrective glasses about two months after surgery. The prognosis is good, and the patient's vision is vastly improved. For the older adult this can mean the difference between social isolation and a meaningful, independent life.

GLAUCOMA

Glaucoma is responsible for blindness in one out of every seven persons, and it is estimated that 1 million Americans have this disease and do not realize it. If glaucoma is diagnosed early enough, however, it can be treated and the chance of blindness eliminated. Thus, the importance of regular eye examinations by the ophthalmologist cannot be overemphasized.

Although the exact cause of glaucoma is unknown, we do know that it involves an increase in the fluid pressure within the eye. The eye normally produces a fluid called aqueous humor, which drains back into the circulatory system through an angle between the iris and cornea. When there is an obstruction or narrowing of this angle in the anterior chamber of the eye, the fluid cannot escape and builds up within the eye. Pressure is exerted upon the optic nerve, and the blood supply to the nerve is diminished, causing damage and eventual blindness if the disease is not treated.

Symptoms such as painful, reddened eyes and vomiting may occur suddenly when there is an acute obstruction of the anterior chamber angle. This is called acute glaucoma. However, the most common form of glaucoma in the senior citizen is chronic glaucoma, which is due to a progressive buildup of fluid pressure within the eye. It is called the sneak thief of sight because its symptoms are minor until changes in vision occur. The patient may complain that his glasses need to be changed, or he may continually wipe his lenses in an effort to correct blurred vision. Vague complaints of headaches, tearing eyes, or difficulty adjusting to the dark are common. Seeing halos around lights is a frequent complaint. Loss of side vision is an early symptom of the disease, but patients are usually unaware of the loss until it becomes severe. Pedestrian accidents in which the person walks into the flow of oncoming traffic may be due to the absence of side vision. Central vision in chronic glaucoma is not lost until the disease is quite advanced.

Diagnosis is made by measuring the amount of pressure within the eye with an instrument called a tonometer. An intraocular reading of 24 mm of mercury or above usually indicates a case of glaucoma. A family history of glaucoma is significant. The angle of the anterior chamber of the eye is examined with a special machine called a gonioscope. The ophthalmologist will perform a complete eye examination to determine the extent of optic nerve damage.

Once the condition has been diagnosed, there is a tendency for the patient to think that blindness is inevitable. Caught in time, however, glaucoma will respond to prompt, continuous treatment that can prevent further complications. Treatment usually involves the prescription of medications called miotics, which constrict the pupil, thereby widening the angle and enabling proper drainage to take place. The patient administers his medications, which are usually in the form of eye drops, every day, just as the diabetic must take insulin every day. The patient and his family need to be instructed on the proper procedure for instilling eye drops. If the patient says he notices an improvement in sight, it is no reason for him to avoid instilling his eye drops. He needs to understand the importance of daily eye medication under all circumstances.

The physician will also discuss the signs of allergic reactions to the drugs with the patient. Oral medications that tend to decrease the rate of formation of aqueous humor may also be ordered. Of course, the patient should continue to have regular eye examinations by the ophthalmologist.

If the use of medication does not relieve intraocular pressure, surgery will be performed. The operation, called an iridectomy, leaves a permanent opening that allows the drainage of aqueous humor.

Although glaucoma cannot be cured, it can be controlled. The patient and his family need to be aware of those activities that tend to increase intraocular pressure and plan daily routines that avoid these activities. Regular bowel habits are important. Constipation should be avoided or treated promptly, since straining to defecate can cause increased pressure. Precautions should be taken to avoid the possibility of an upper respiratory infection, which would result in coughs and sneezes. No medication should be used without the ophthalmologist's permission. Patented cold medicines are especially dangerous to the glaucoma patient, because they contain decongestants, which cause vasoconstriction. The prescribed eye medication should not be allowed to be depleted. An extra supply should be properly labeled and stored in a safe place.

Anxiety and emotional stress can contribute to an increase in intraocular pressure, and situations that precipitate worry, anger, or excitement should be avoided as much as possible. Excessive intake of fluid at one time and tight constricting clothing can also cause a rise in pressure. The ophthalmologist will advise the patient concerning the use of sunglasses. In some cases continuous use of sunglasses or remaining in a darkened room for a long period of time may create untoward effects. Activities that contribute to eye fatigue or strain should be avoided.

The patient will be advised to carry a card or wear a medi-bracelet stating that he has glaucoma. In the event of an accident or sudden illness, the prescribed therapy can then be carried out without delay. If the patient moves away from home, he should request that all medical records be transferred to the new ophthalmologist.

The patient and his family should know that cheating on the physician's orders can be very dangerous. If the patient follows directions, his chances of maintaining existing eyesight are very good. Adjusting to minor changes in the daily routine is not a high price to pay for a most precious possession—sight.

THE DEPRESSED AND SUICIDAL PATIENT

Psychologically, the elderly person may go through periods of depression. These periods can be most disturbing to the individual as well as to his family. Although everyone, no matter what age, has highs and lows in his emotional life, the lows may recur more frequently among the elderly. These lows may be caused by the loss of one's spouse, loved ones, friends. Social isolation, waning energy, the awareness of mortality, physical adjustments associated with aging—all are contributing factors to these periods of depression. Another cause may be a psychotic reaction or depression associated with confusion and disorientation as a result of decreased blood flow through cerebral arteriosclerotic vessels. Prolonged grief, too, may lead to severe depression. For those who have had difficulty in coping with these feelings and resolving conflicts in the past, the states of depression become more difficult to handle as time goes on.

Marked depression is characterized by loss of appetite and weight, constipation, and altered sleeping patterns—the patient may awaken between 2:00 and 3:00 A.M. and be unable to return to sleep. He may lose all interest in his surroundings and complain of many nonspecific physical problems. Hopefully, the family and patient will seek professional help through the family physician, who will direct the patient to the local mental health center or a psychiatrist for additional help. Treatment is aimed at helping the patient to regain his self-esteem and develop the ability to cope with the causes of the depression. Antidepressive drugs and electroconvulsive therapy may be ordered in conjunction with psychotherapy.

If the states of depression become pronounced and go untreated, the elderly person may decide that the only way out is suicide. The suicide rate for white men reaches its peak when they are in their eighties. The peak for white women is in middle life (forty-five to fifty-five). The suicide rate for nonwhites is low and reaches its peak at twenty-five to thirty-four years of age. Thus, the threat of suicide is especially serious among older white males. Depression is present in 80 percent of those who consider or attempt suicide. Should an unsuccessful suicide attempt occur, a second try is quite probable. The aged are serious in their attempts to end it all, for they see no other way out. The person may threaten suicide or confide that he wishes he were dead. These comments should never be taken lightly and should be reported to the physician immediately. If the threat is unheeded, it may be carried out in a variety of ways. Usually, once the decision has been reached, the patient's behavior changes—he becomes less depressed. This change is misleading, since the individual appears to be improving. In reality, he is less depressed because he has decided how to correct his situation. All behavior changes must be reported to the physician, and the nurse must observe the patient carefully.

Suicide is apt to occur at a time of personal crisis for the depressed person. Bereavement, physical illness, diagnosis of a disease with an uncertain prognosis can all be predisposing factors for a suicide attempt. Loneliness is a particular problem, for it causes a lowered self-esteem and a feeling of lack of worth. It is estimated that 10 to 20 percent of the aged population live in social isolation. Gerontologists have begun to discuss and define a retirement syndrome of severe depression, which often follows the termination of gainful employment.

In periods of acute stress or personal crisis, the aged person needs to be able to turn to someone who understands and can help him. Many communities have a telephone service that enables the senior citizen to talk with a professional counselor. This service, which may have one of many names such as Help, Prevention, or Life Line, is usually sponsored by a mental health clinic, a hospital, or some other mental health agency. In addition to receiving immediate crisis counseling, the individual can make appointments and obtain referrals for short- and long-term therapy.

For a detailed discussion of suicide refer to a standard psychiatric nursing text.

THE DISORIENTED AND CONFUSED PATIENT

For many years the term "senile" has been used to describe the elderly person who displays unusual behavior. To the general public, this catchall word has been automatically associated with the aging process. Senility is thought of as a dreaded, inevitable consequence of aging. We know that this is not correct. The chronic, irreversible deterioration of mental capabilities, caused in part by brain degeneration, is more appropriately called chronic brain disorder rather than senility. It has been found that this disorder is also influenced by personality patterns built up during a lifetime. The well-adjusted, mature adult who is emotionally and intellectually active is less likely to display the changes in behavior associated with the disease than the person whose life-style has been one of insecurity and rigidity.

Research has shown that the most common cause of progressive permanent brain damage in the elderly results from the presence of cerebral vascular disease. The arteries carying oxygen-laden blood to the brain become smaller in size due to arteriosclerosis. Therefore, the oxygen supply to a part of the brain is decreased, causing the gradual death of local nerve tissue. As the disease progresses, larger areas of the brain are affected. The process is usually gradual, and symptoms depend on the extent of the brain damage. The terms "senility," "senile brain disease," and "organic brain syndrome" all describe this most perplexing condition.

Symptoms of the disease usually occur after the age of sixty. Family members are generally not aware of the onset of symptoms. In the beginning there is a lapse of memory for recent events, which the patient handles quite well. He merely makes up a story to compensate for the memory loss. Personality characteristics that have developed through the years will tend to be exaggerated. For example, the woman who kept paper bags because "you never know when you'll need one" will hoard them in a secret place by the hundreds. The stern elderly man will be overly gruff and sometimes nasty to family members.

Symptoms tend to be aggravated by stress, both physical and psychological. If the older person is not under stress, he may have periods when he is mentally alert and behaves in a normal manner. A good day may be followed by a day when confusion and disorientation appear. As brain deterioration progresses, the symptoms are also magnified. Memory gaps become more frequent, and the individual is no longer able to compensate by storytelling. Although recent events are foggy or completely blotted out in the person's mind, he is able to recall the events of the past in great detail. He will tell and retell of situations that occurred fifty years ago as if they had happened yesterday. Social and intellectual interests are reduced, and the person turns inward, living more and more in the past. The patient's interest in others now turns to interest in himself, his physical symptoms, and his bodily functions.

The patient's disorientation regarding time (including the hour, day, month, and year), place, and relationships (such as his relationship to a daughter or son) can be a real problem for the family to handle. He may believe that he is just visiting friends for the day and wander out of his own home. Many of these disoriented people are luckily found by police and returned home, provided they are carrying identification. However, some are not as fortunate. Along with confusion and disorientation, there is a tendency for mood changes, which can be quite abrupt. The calm, quiet, elderly woman can suddenly burst into tears or become belligerent and demanding, seemingly without sufficient cause. Extreme irritability, verbal expressions of hostility, or actual temper tantrums may be triggered by an insignificant event. Failing eyesight and hearing loss magnify problems for older persons who are confused and disoriented. Their ability to cope with changes in routine and any other deviations from the known is greatly reduced. They are disturbed by even slight variations in family life patterns. Rearranged furniture, changes in meal schedules, and unknown visitors are tolerated poorly if at all. Thinking processes are also impaired, and errors in their judgment, particularly in financial matters, may lead to exploitation of the elderly.

Sleeping patterns may include short periods of sleep at night, and confusion may be more prevalent at night. Because of insomnia the confused person may wander aimlessly about during the early morning hours. Unstable gait and posture, slowed reflexes and movements, and poor eyesight contribute to a high incidence of accidents among those who do this. If possible, the older person's bedroom should be located on the ground floor to avoid the possibility of his falling down a flight of steps.

Deterioration may also be shown by the patient's careless physical appearance and poor personal habits. He may exhibit socially unacceptable behavior, such as using obscene language, acting out sexual impulses, or disrobing.

The physician will base his diagnosis on evidence of an intellectual decline that is progressive and chronic in character. Along with the family's description of the gradual onset and progression of symptoms, the physician will utilize tests to determine the patient's ability to remember and to do abstract reasoning. Other disease processes such as brain tumors will be ruled out by performing a lumbar puncture and electroencephalogram. The possibility of functional mental disorders will also need to be eliminated.

Treatment will depend on the symptoms displayed. Medications such as vasodilators, which help to increase the blood supply to brain tissue, may be ordered. Tranquilizers may also be indicated.

Home Care

The family will be encouraged to care for the elderly person at home as long as possible. A familiar environment helps to minimize confusion and disorientation, provided the environment is kept fairly stable. Since the patient does not tolerate change very well, the family needs to understand why changes in routine should be avoided. The family may need help in planning an appropriate schedule to accommodate the needs of both the patient and the other family members. The schedule should allow for periods of rest and outdoor physical activity for the patient if possible. Without this proper balance, he will revert to dozing in a chair during the day, followed by nighttime insomnia. This pattern is progressively harder to break as the days go by. Physical activity such as walking out of doors will help to give the patient a sense of well-being and will exercise joints and muscles, which will become stiff if they are not used. Fresh air and exercise during the day can be just what is needed to cure insomnia.

Good nutrition is essential for all elderly persons and especially for the disoriented and confused. The patient will require extra time to eat, and his table manners may not be the best. He is most likely to eat those foods that have been a part of his diet throughout the years. The cook in the family should be cautioned against trying out a new dish that is unfamiliar to the patient. He may well reject the entire meal. Snacks in between meals and especially before bedtime are helpful.

The patient should perform activities of daily living as long as possible with encouragement from his family. The older person should not be permitted to leave nightclothes on during the day, but should dress properly in daytime wear. The family will need to assist in activities of daily living when indicated.

Since the patient may not always be aware of safety precautions, other members of the family must assume increasing responsibilities. The confused, disoriented smoker can be a real hazard to others.

Perhaps the most critical problem the family faces in caring for the confused person is that of coping with his behavior patterns and the communication difficulties. He will need to be oriented to time, place, and persons as necessary—perhaps several times a day. When speaking to him, family members should use a calm approach. Their speech should be slow and distinct, and they should face the elderly person directly. If they display impatience or irritation, the patient's symptoms will tend to increase. Caring for the disoriented and confused at home can be a most frustrating experience.

As deterioration progresses, the physician may suggest that the family have assistance from a public health nurse in caring for the patient. In addition to assisting with physical care, the nurse will help in formulating a realistic schedule to accommodate the patient's increasing mental deterioration. The nurse provides an opportunity for family members to verbalize their feelings of frustration, irritation, and helplessness in coping with the everyday problems.

The effects of caring for the confused person on the total family unit will need to be evaluated by the physician. When it is determined and agreed that the patient's condition warrants a transfer to an institution, necessary arrangements will be made. Unfortunately, because there is a lack of suitable facilities for this type of patient, many are hospitalized in institutions for the mentally ill. This is a difficult decision for the family to make and requires considerable emotional support on the part of the physician and the nursing personnel.

Institutional Care

The patient's initial reaction following transfer to the health care institution is usually characterized by an aggravation of the behavior patterns previously established. Since he has difficulty tolerating any change, the transfer from a familiar setting to a whole new environment will be a shock. The patient who was hostile at home may now exhibit more aggressive and mistrusting behavior. Another patient, whose pattern at home was one of dependency, may demonstrate childlike behavior or complete withdrawal. The family members may blame themselves for an increase in symptoms, which appear to be caused by placing the patient in an institution, and they will need assistance from the staff in understanding why these changes, sometimes drastic, have occurred.

The nurse, realizing the patient's difficulty in adjusting to new surroundings, will develop a nursing care plan that will help the patient through this initial phase. There are several important considerations, which have to do with the nurse's attitude toward the patient. The plan will revolve around one essential concept—that of respect for the patient's inherent worth. Although he is confused and disoriented, the patient should be treated with dignity as another member of humanity. Although bizarre behavior may now be in evidence, the nurse realizes that the patient was once a contributing member of society and that his past achievements are worthy of respect. Calling the patient familiar names such as Pop or Mom is degrading to the patient. The use of his proper name and title will help him to maintain his dignity and self-respect. In developing the care plan, the nurse should find out as much as she can about the patient's past activities. The family, acting as resource persons, can give valuable information on such things as his likes and dislikes, his ability to perform activities of daily living, his behavior patterns, and events that tend to aggravate his behavior. If the patient was accustomed to a bedroom of his own, sharing a room with others can add to his confusion and present problems in his adjusting to roommates. The nurse should encourage the family to relate any other special information about the patient that would be helpful in developing an individualized plan of care.

The nursing care plan will include orienting the patient to his new surroundings—his room, the bathroom, recreation area, dining area, etc. This general orientation will need to be repeated due to the patient's memory lapses. The strange environment can, however, be made less foreign if the patient is allowed to bring some cherished possessions with him. If these items are placed around his room or bed area, they can help in his orientation, especially if the patient shares a room with others. One bed unit in a nursing home can look like any other to the confused patient. The treasures from home help to personalize his new environment. Women patients should be permitted to carry their pocketbooks. This provides a place where articles can be stored—a private spot. The men will want to carry their wallets, and these serve the same purpose—giving the patient a sense of identity. The lack of privacy may be severely felt by the patient who has lived alone or has had his own bedroom. The pocketbook, wallet, and other cherished items may be the only links that are left with the former private life. Dressing in clothing from home rather than in hospital wear helps the patient to maintain his individual identity.

In addition to an orientation to place, the patient will need help in establishing time. In many institutions clocks with large readable dials are placed in convenient locations throughout the patient areas. Some patients may want to wear a wristwatch. The nurse can remind them to wind the watch and check its accuracy. Newspapers and current magazines assist in orienting the patient to the date, month, and year. Of course, calendars that are strategically placed and large enough for easy reading also help. In areas where the seasons change, calendars with appropriate scenes for each month provide visual help.

Nursing personnel will assist the patient in getting to know the people surrounding him—patients as well as the staff of the unit. Initially, the patient may become more confused because of the changes in staff from one shift to another. In fact, he may never fully adjust to the coming and going of favorite staff members. Just as helping the patient to adjust to place and time requires considerable repetition, repetition is necessary to orient him to other residents and staff. It takes considerable patience on the part of the nursing personnel to answer the same question for the twentieth time. An abrupt remark such as, "Mrs. Johnson, you know I just told you where the recreation room is," only creates more confusion, more forgetfulness, and most of all, a feeling of helplessness and loneliness.

During the patient's initial period of adjustment, the nursing personnel may have to assume more responsibility for his activities of daily living. This necessity will decrease as he begins to function in his new environment. However, the nurse will need to remind him to perform such activities. Expert care is necessary to prevent deformities and other medical problems. Even though the patient is disoriented and confused, the nurse should explain any treatment before she administers it, just as she does for the nonconfused patient.

During this initial phase of care, the nursing personnel should observe the emerging patterns of behavior and, through nursing staff conferences, begin to develop plans for coping with the type of behavior manifested. Some of the most common patterns include aggression, mistrust, regression, withdrawal, and hostility.

If, after a period of time, the patient has not settled in and adjusted to his new environment, the family members and nursing staff may become impatient. This attitude, which is readily felt by the patient, does not help to make him feel wanted and secure. In fact, as a result of it, he may take even longer to learn to trust the staff. He may accuse his nurse of stealing his wallet or hiding his dentures, when in reality he has forgotten where he has placed them. Fortunately, the patient usually misplaces them in one or two familiar spots. The nurse should note the location of lost items in the care plan so everyone will know where to look for lost objects. Nurses can be frustrated by the patient's accusations and his forgetfulness. Remember that this behavior is a symptom of the patient's organic disease. Patience and understanding are essential if the patient is to feel secure and wanted.

Occasionally, the patient will mistake the nurse for someone whom he intensely dislikes. He may be exceedingly hostile toward the nurse—refusing to eat the food she brings, refusing medications, ignoring her altogether. The nurse should remind the patient of her name, title, and function. If such an approach proves futile, it is best for the patient to be reassigned to another staff member. Conversely, patients may mistake nursing personnel for a beloved member of their family—daughter, son, spouse, or parent. Again the nurse should tell the patient exactly who she is. This will have to be done many, many times because of the patient's difficulty in remembering.

Nurses who work in institutions for the confused and disoriented elderly patient have commented that these people frequently exhibit child-like behavior. However, since people will behave very much as they are treated and in the way they are expected to behave, patients who present a pattern of childlike behavior should *not* be treated like children. They should be approached as mature adults who can understand simple, clear explanations and requests.

Regression is a common problem and may be manifested in a variety of behaviors, two common manifestations being depression and incontinence of bowel and bladder. The tearful and depressed geriatric patient needs reassurance, warmth, and love, which are best conveyed by putting your arms around the patient and offering him comfort and understanding.

Bladder and bowel incontinence can be avoided by reminding the patient where the bathroom is and when to use this facility. Regular toileting can eliminate the need for diapers, prevent decubitus formation, and eliminate the odor of urine and feces. Furthermore, successful toileting will increase the patient's self-esteem and reduce his embarrassment over accidents.

The withdrawn patient will remain alone and aloof from others. He has little or no interest in his surroundings and is usually unkempt and uninterested in his personal appearance and hygiene. The nurse must remind the patient to perform activities of daily living and may have to assume responsibility for completing them.

In many psychiatric institutions a technique known as Remotivation has been helpful in stimulating withdrawn and confused individuals to communicate with others. This simple group interaction is usually conducted by the psychiatric aide, who has been trained in the procedure. Remotivation is an excellent method for reaching a group of elderly institutionalized persons and maintaining and/or increasing their interest in life. Special training courses to prepare remotivation leaders are offered in various locations in the United States. These brief but intense courses may be offered at regional centers or at a nearby hospital where the technique is utilized. Further information can be obtained from American Psychiatric Association, 1700 Eighteenth Street, N.W., Washington, D. C. 20009.

Patients may be terrified by illusions and/or hallucinations. Their fears may be calmed by giving them simple reassurance and offering them protection and comfort. The nurse should not hesitate to comfort the patient by means of touching—stroking his head, holding his hand, placing arms around the shoulders. Although the hallucination is very realistic to the patient, the nurse should not acknowledge something she does not see. The nurse should never go along with the patient merely to humor him. Such a deception is childlike and will not reassure or comfort him.

Illusions frequently take the form of the patient's mistaking one person for another. For example, the patient may mistake a son for his father. The patient must always be told the true identity of the person. The illusion may subside, so that the patient will recognize the person himself. It is not unusual for the patient to say at a later date, "I was confused about you, Bob. I thought you were my father, but of course he's been dead for years." If the nurse plays games and pretends to see or hear something the patient falsely perceives, she does not help the patient to maintain contact with reality and may even increase his confusion and disorientation.

Some patients may exhibit behavior that is considered socially unacceptable. Examples would be masturbation, exposure of the genitalia, swearing and offensive language, and sexual overtures to the nurses (male and female). Patients are often ostracized for such behavior. Unfortunately sometimes being locked in their rooms and left alone. A variety of techniques can be utilized to deal with this kind of behavior. One of the most effective is meaningful, diversional activity. The staff should also attempt to find reasons underlying the patient's behavior. For example, is a female patient masturbating, or does she have a physical problem, such as senile vaginitis, that is causing irritation and itching?

The physician may order tranquilizing drugs for the patient who exhibits bizarre behavior. The nursing staff should observe the effects of drug therapy and report any untoward effects to the physician. A tranquilizer should not render a patient insensible. Nor are tranquilizers substitutes for excellent nursing care.

The confused and disoriented patient will spend the rest of his life in the institution. The nursing personnel's goal should be to make his remaining years as happy and meaningful as possible.

There is usually a direct correlation between the length of the patient's stay and the frequency of the family's visits. The longer the stay, the fewer the visits. The nurse will find this hard to accept and may feel that the family is cruel and unkind. However, these feelings should never be revealed to the patient. It is sad but true that for the patient who lives to be very old, the nursing home staff ultimately becomes his substitute family—loving him, comforting him, and finally mourning him.

STUDY QUESTION

The Hanleys, who are both in their eighties, have been married for fifty-five years and now live with their only daughter and her husband. Mrs. Hanley has been able to help her daughter keep house for some time. She does not perform physically exhausting work, but says, "My specialty is starting meals, dusting, and doing the dishes." More than that, she sees to Mr. Hanley's needs. He has become forgetful lately, needs to be reminded to go to the bathroom, and is sometimes confused. Mr. Hanley talks only with his wife and does not communicate with the others in the household. He rarely goes out, except to pick the newspaper up off the front steps. A considerable portion of his day is spent sleeping, and he is restless and suffers insomnia at night.

For some time Mrs. Hanley has been complaining about poor vision. Finally, her daughter took a day off from her job and took Mrs. Hanley to the ophthalmologist. The physician diagnosed Mrs. Hanley's problem as bilateral senile cataracts and advised immediate surgery.

When the two women arrived home, Mrs. Hanley, her daughter, and her son-in-law held a family conference to discuss their problems, and asked you, their neighbor, to help them find some solutions. They had the following problems. What are some possible solutions?

a. Both the daughter and her husband have to work in order to maintain their economic status, which is rather low. What should they do about Mr. Hanley, who needs to have someone with him constantly?

b. Who will care for Mr. and Mrs. Hanley when she comes home from the hospital?

c. They have no hospitalization. Will Medicare pay for the doctor, hospital, and eyeglasses?

BIBLIOGRAPHY

Anderson, Helen. *Newton's Geriatric Nursing.* 5th ed. Saint Louis: C. V. Mosby, 1971.

Beeson, Paul, and McDermott, Walsh, eds. *Textbook of Medicine.* 12th ed. Philadelphia: W. B. Saunders, 1967.

Brunner, Lillian; Emerson, Charles; Ferguson, Kraeer; and Suddarth, Doris. *Textbook of Medical-Surgical Nursing.* 2nd ed. Philadelphia: J. B. Lippincott, 1970.

Carroll, Bettie. "Fingers to Toes." *American Journal of Nursing,* March 1971, p. 550.

Cooper, I. S. *Parkinsonism—A Handbook for Patients and Their Families.* New York: American Parkinson Disease Association, 1966.

Crawford, Annie Laurie, and Buchanan, Barbara Boring. *Psychiatric Nursing, A Basic Manual.* 2nd ed. Philadelphia: F. A. Davis, 1966.

Davis, Robert. "Psychologic Aspects of Geriatric Nursing." *American Journal of Nursing,* April 1968, pp. 802–804.

"Eating and Nutrition in Parkinson's Disease and Syndrome," in the series of pamphlets *Clinical Insights into Parkinson's Disease.* Norwich, N.Y.: Eaton Laboratories, 1970.

Fangman, Anne, and O'Malley, William. "L-dopa and the Patient with Parkinson's Disease." *American Journal of Nursing,* July 1969, p. 1455.

Frenay, Sister Agnes Clare, and Pierce, Gloria. "The Climate of Care for a Geriatric Patient." *American Journal of Nursing,* September 1971, pp. 1747–1750.

Gage, Frances Boland. "Suicide in the Aged." *American Journal of Nursing,* November 1971, p. 2153.

"Guide to Early Recognition of Parkinson's Disease and Syndrome," in the series of pamphlets *Clinical Insights into Parkinson's Disease.* Norwich, N.Y.: Eaton Laboratories, 1970.

Hahn, Aloyse. "It's Tough to Be Old." *American Journal of Nursing,* August 1970, pp. 1698–1699.

Hays, Joyce Sanhammer, and Larson, Kenneth. *Interacting with Patients.* New York: Macmillan, 1968.

Hofling, Charles H.; Leininger, Madeleine M.; and Bregg, Elizabeth A. *Basic Psychiatric Concepts in Nursing.* 2nd ed. Philadelphia: J. B. Lippincott, 1967.

Jaeger, Dorothea, and Simmons, Leo. *The Aged Ill—Coping with Problems of Geriatric Care.* New York: Appleton-Century-Crofts, 1970.

Johnston, Mabyl. *Mental Health and Mental Illness.* Philadelphia: J. B. Lippincott, 1971.

Jourard, Sidney. "Suicide—The Invitation to Die." *American Journal of Nursing,* February 1970, p. 269.

Let Your Light So Shine. Nutley, N.J.: Roche Laboratories.

Public Health Service and National Institutes of Health, *Parkinson's Disease—Hope Through Research.* Washington, D.C.: U.S. Government Printing Office, 1971.

Robinson, Alice. *Remotivation Technique.* Washington, D.C.: American Psychiatric Association and Smith Kline French Labs Remotivation Project.

Rossman, Isodore. *Clinical Geriatrics*. Philadelphia: J. B. Lippincott, 1968.

Seeman, Bernard. *Your Sight*. Boston: Little, Brown, 1968.

Sloane, Albert E. *So You Have Cataracts*. Springfield, Ill.: Charles C Thomas, 1970.

Smith, Dorothy; Germain, Carol; and Gips, Claudia. *Care of the Adult Patient*. 3rd ed. Philadelphia: J. B. Lippincott, 1971.

"Treatment of Adverse Reactions to DOPAR," in the series of pamphlets *Clinical Insights into Parkinson's Disease*. Norwich, N.Y.: Eaton Laboratories, 1970.

Veirs, Everett R. *So You Have Glaucoma*. 2nd ed. New York: Grune & Stratton, 1970.

U.S., Department of Health, Education, and Welfare, *Working with Older People—A Guide to Practice*, vol. 4, *Clinical Aspects of Aging*, Austin B. Chinn, ed. Washington, D.C.: U.S. Government Printing Office, 1971.

10

Restorative Nursing of Patients with Diseases of the Circulatory-Respiratory Systems

Recent advances in medical research and technology have helped to add years to the average life-span. Unfortunately, the incidence of cerebral vascular disease also increases as years are added to our lives. In fact, cerebral vascular disease is the third leading cause of hospitalization for those who are sixty-five or over. According to the latest available statistics, 1.6 million Americans are stroke victims, and each year approximately 5 million will suffer from their first attack. Should they survive, the likelihood of their experiencing a recurrence is great. Each year cerebral vascular disease accounts for 12 percent of all deaths among the elderly. It ranks third after heart disease and cancer as a leading cause of death in the United States.

Cerebral vascular disease occurs when circulation of blood within the brain is impaired, causing a reduction in the nourishment going to surrounding brain tissue. This cutting off of adequate nourishment results in death of brain cells and malfunctioning of the central nervous system. Arteriosclerosis and hypertension both contribute to these conditions.

CEREBRAL VASCULAR ACCIDENT

One of the most common cerebral vascular diseases among senior citizens is the cerebral vascular accident, or stroke. There are four major causes, all of which result in a lack of blood supply to cerebral tissue: (1) A blood clot, or thrombus, may form in an artery or vein, resulting in partial or total obstruction of blood flow. Also, a traveling clot, or embolus, from another part of the body may find its way to the cerebral vessel and lodge there. (2) If the wall of a cerebral blood vessel is weakened and the blood pressure is increased, there may be a "blow out," or rupture, of the weak artery. Hemorrhage results, with blood flowing out into surrounding tissue. (3) Tumors or clots outside the vessel may cause pressure, which compresses the walls of the blood vessel and closes off the blood flow. (4) Spasms or contractions of the muscles of the vessel wall may close off the normal flow of blood through the opening. Arteriosclerosis also contributes to a narrowing of the opening through which the blood flows.

Although the onset of an acute attack is sudden, there are certain signs that may identify the stroke-prone person before the acute symptoms appear. Techniques in preventive medicine are geared toward detecting these potential patients and instituting measures to help prevent the initial attack from occurring. Two of the signs—hypertension and arteriosclerosis —have already been mentioned. Other danger signals are a history of heart disease, excess weight, cigarette smoking (particularly in men), and high blood cholesterol.

Some patients may exhibit symptoms indicating that "mini" strokes have occurred. The symptoms are short-lived, and the patient may be able to conceal them, so that they may go unnoticed. Slurred speech, blurred vision, dizziness, numbness of hands and fingers, and some mental confusion may be the only symptoms. They may be caused by cerebral ischemia, or a temporarily diminished blood supply to small areas of brain tissue. Unfortunately, if these mini strokes go untreated, they may one day result in a cerebral vascular accident sufficient in size to present major symptoms. The symptoms will depend on the extent and location of the brain damage as well as the cause. If a large area of brain tissue is affected, death may be immediate. The attack may come without warning, or it may be preceded by vague complaints of fatigue, headache, and mini-stroke symptoms. Gradual paralysis of one side of the body, or hemiplegia, and sensory difficulties may appear over a period of several hours. The patient may be conscious or comatose. If hemiplegia occurs, the patient will show evidence of weakness on one side of his body. His facial muscles will also be affected, and his mouth will droop on the affected side. Slurred speech, labored deep respirations, a flushed face, and incontinence are additional symptoms.

Immediate care of the patient demonstrating these symptoms requires the maintenance of an unobstructed airway. To accomplish this, any constricting clothing should be removed and the patient's head turned to the side so that secretions can drain from the side of the mouth. Since an acute medical emergency exists, the patient is usually admitted to the intensive care unit of the hospital, where treatment is based on life-saving measures.

Confirmation of the diagnosis will be obtained from the physical examination and studies of the cerebrospinal fluid, obtained by means of a lumbar puncture. Skull X rays, an electroencephalogram, and electrocardiogram readings will assist the physician in evaluating the patient's condition. Cerebral angiography, the technique of injecting a radiopaque substance into the arteries supplying blood to the brain, will show upon X ray the existence of clots that are shutting off the flow of blood and the specific areas of injury. If the area is surgically accessible, the surgeon may open the artery and remove the obstructing clot. Many patients experiencing mini strokes show evidence of thrombi in the neck arteries supplying blood to the brain, and surgical removal of the obstruction can prevent the inevitable cerebral vascular accident.

Although surgery is indicated in some cases, it is not always possible, and a large percentage of patients will not benefit from such treatment. The initial therapy for these patients will be aimed first of all at saving their life and at limiting the amount of brain damage. The rehabilitation program will then be directed at reducing deformity and disability. The prevention of recurrences is another major treatment goal. The principles already covered in Chapter 6 apply to the patient recovering from a cerebral vascular accident. The active rehabilitative program usually begins immediately after the patient's neurological symptoms stabilize. Two symptoms —aphasia and hemiplegia—require special rehabilitation considerations.

Aphasia

One of man's unique abilities is that of communicating his thoughts to others through speech and writing. This is a complicated process involving the ability of the body to receive messages from the surrounding environment, analyze them, formulate a response, and then transmit the response in the form of a gesture or a spoken or written word. The ability to communicate is controlled by a center located in the left hemisphere of the brain. Those patients who have hemiplegia of the right side of the body usually experience some difficulty in communicating. When this occurs, the patient's symptom is known as aphasia.

Aphasia is classified according to whether the patient has difficulty in taking in or interpreting stimuli from outside the body or in responding by means of spoken or written language. In *receptive aphasia* the problem is in the receiving of external stimuli. The patient may have difficulty in recognizing objects or in understanding what is said or what he reads. With *expressive aphasia,* the inability to respond to external stimuli, the patient has difficulty in making his thoughts and wishes known to others by means of speech, gestures, or writing. Most aphasic patients will have both receptive and expressive symptoms. When this occurs, the term *mixed aphasia* is used.

Speech therapy should be initiated early in the patient's recovery program. The speech pathologist, commonly called a speech therapist, is a member of the rehabilitation team and his special abilities enable him to treat a variety of speech disorders. The speech pathologist will institute measures that will help the patient to fully utilize his remaining communicating skills and to improve the accuracy and consistency of his performance. The particular measures will depend on the type of aphasia, and speech therapy sessions will be highly individualized to suit the patient's abilities and needs. As the damaged portion of the brain heals, the patient's ability to communicate through language, writing, and gestures will improve. The therapist will adjust the speech therapy program as these changes occur, so that hopefully the patient will be able to fully utilize his communication potential.

Patients' reactions to difficulties in communication are as varied as the individuals themselves. Certainly, they experience great frustration and depression. For those who have been very verbal prior to the cerebral vascular accident, coping with aphasia can be extremely difficult. The patient may react by isolating himself from others, thereby eliminating the need to communicate. He may show complete lack of interest in his surroundings as well as symptoms of severe depression. All his energies are focused on his own problems, allowing him little or no time to be concerned about others. The family may react negatively to the patient's self-centeredness, and they should be made aware of his inner turmoil. The nurse plays a vital role in helping the patient and his family through this very trying time. The nurse's attitude in handling communication difficulties can either stimulate or retard the therapy process. Remember that the patient's ability to recover his communicating skills may not be directly linked to his ability to ambulate or perform activities of daily living. These functions are independent of communication, and it usually takes longer for language skills to return than it does for physical ones.

Each patient's symptoms and resulting communication problems will vary according to the extent and area of brain damage. Generally, there will be some intellectual impairment. Memory of recent events may be poor, although past events are usually remembered quite well. Some families may begin to associate the patient's aphasia with mental deterioration and treat him like a child. This raises the patient's frustration level and contributes to his feeling of total helplessness. The family needs to know that the patient is not mentally incompetent and that he should be treated as a mature and intelligent adult.

The patient may be able to understand what is being said to him and know what he wants to say in response, but words don't come out the way he wants. He may use the word "chair" for "table" or confuse gestures by shaking his head to indicate no when he really means yes. Some patients may lose the names of objects. They may be able to speak in sentences but unable to remember the noun to complete the thought. Thus, for example, a patient might say, "Please give me the . . . . You know what I mean," rather than "Please give me the bedpan." This situation can be most frustrating for both the patient and the nurse and may result in a guessing game unless a system of communication is established.

One way of handling the situation is for the nurse to give the patient cue cards with pictures of frequently used items on them. The name of the object is written below each picture. If necessary, the patient can point to the item he needs. The nurse then names the object, which helps the patient to relearn the word. The nursing care plan should indicate the progress the patient is making in recognizing these words. In some instances the patient can write even though he can't speak, in which case a small chalkboard or magic slate can be used for communication between the nurse and patient. The nurse may find that the patient is able to repeat words that are said but has great difficulty in naming objects without help.

Some patients may recite poems, count, and use common phrases such as "Good Morning," "How are you?" but be unable to go beyond this point in conversation. This recitation of familiar words or phrases is called *automatic or primitive language*. Although the patient is unable to express his thoughts and ideas in original sentences, he may be able to speak in the above manner, which can be misleading to the family members, who consider these automatic language outbursts as signs of recovery. Usually, if the patient is asked to repeat a phrase, he is inconsistent, and he may not be able to repeat what he has just said.

Bilingual patients usually find it easier to use their native language rather than the acquired language. For example, the patient who was born and raised in Italy will tend to recover Italian words first, rather than English words.

In some instances the patient's conversation will be so garbled that it cannot be understood. Sounds are put together, but the results are not actual words. Rather they are something that sounds like double-talk. The patient is unable to control this and may or may not be aware of his difficulty.

Although the speech disturbances of patients with aphasia vary widely, there are some basic rules the nursing staff must employ in helping these patients to cope with their problems in communicating. If the aphasic patient is to learn to utilize his communication potential, attention must be given to his ability to see and hear properly. The patient may not recognize relatives or visitors because he doesn't have his glasses, or he may not respond to the nurse's question because he can't hear. The nurse should encourage the patient to wear his eyeglasses or his hearing aid. Also poorly fitting dentures or lack of teeth can vastly reduce the patient's ability to speak in an understandable way. Eyeglasses, hearing aids, and dentures may be some of the essential elements in helping the patient compensate for losses in communication.

Since nursing personnel spend the major part of each day with the patient, they are in a unique position to encourage speech. Emphasis should be placed on fostering speech rather than anticipating the patient's needs. If the patient doesn't have to speak, he may not make the necessary effort. Feelings of inadequacy will result, and the motivation to speak will be lost. When addressing the patient, the nurse should speak slowly and distinctly, face the patient directly, and speak to his unaffected side if possible. Although the reason is not completely understood, addressing the patient's unaffected side helps to increase his comprehension. Short, simple sentences are easier for the patient to understand than long, complex sentences incorporating more than one thought.

Conversation should be geared to present events that are occurring in the patient's immediate surroundings. Abstract subjects should be avoided, and the conversation should be limited to familar topics of interest to the patient. It may be difficult for the patient to follow a conversation on a subject with which he is unfamiliar. If the nurse's attitude is that of encouraging speech, ample time must be given for the patient to respond to her questions. Although the experience can be taxing on the nurse's nerves, a calm exterior will help the patient in his struggle to reply. If he detects lack of interest, boredom, or frustration from the nurse's outward appearance, he may give up trying. Remember, the battle is won with small victories along the way. Praise when indicated can be just the tonic to stimulate the patient to try harder. An overly critical attitude can be discouraging to the patient. A happy medium, somewhere between over-protectiveness and nagging, needs to be fostered. The patient must feel accepted and wanted if he is to improve his communication skills. Both the nurse and the family must strive to communicate this feeling verbally and nonverbally.

The patient will have enough problems understanding and/or responding to the conversation around him without having to compete with distractions, such as a blaring radio or television. Therefore, the most conducive atmosphere is one in which there are relatively few distractions. Nursing personnel and family will need to understand that the patient's attention span will be short and that sudden shifts in conversation from one person to another will be difficult for him to follow.

The patient's ability to communicate will fluctuate from day to day and with the time of day. His best speech will probably occur early in the day. As he fatigues, speech will become poorer. Consistency in communication will stabilize as his condition improves. Speech therapy sessions will usually be planned early in the day to take advantage of the best time of the patient's day. Short sessions of five to fifteen minutes per session reap better results than prolonged ones. In rehabilitation team conferences the therapist shares the patient's progress and problems with the other members of the team. The nursing care plan should reflect the progress made during speech therapy sessions, so that proper reinforcement of learning will continue.

The physician may encourage patient participation in speech therapy group sessions. Although these sessions should never be substituted for individual speech therapy treatments, they may be an important addition. The most important advantage of group sessions is that they assist the patient in his social readjustment. The realization that others have similar problems may have a therapeutic effect. Group activities should include those that everyone can perform, since the inability to participate will create feelings of inadequacy, depression, embarrassment—in fact, all those emotions that tear down, rather than build up, self-esteem. One activity that all patients are usually able to participate in is group singing.

The family plays a major role in the patient's progress. The nurse alone cannot create a speech-encouraging climate. Assistance from the family is an essential ingredient. Initially, the family members must understand the patient's problem. They need to know what aphasia is and why the patient may have periods when he cries, becomes angry, or acts withdrawn. The nurse needs to be a good listener. Family members need help too in adjusting to this traumatic situation. In their anxious enthusiasm to help the patient to get better, some relatives and friends will bombard the patient with questions that he is incapable of answering or cannot understand. The patient may react to his inability to perform with anger or tears. At the other extreme, some families provide no opportunity for the patient to communicate, either by speaking, writing, or gesturing.

Family members need to know the helpful hints discussed earlier for achieving and maintaining effective communication with the aphasic patient. The nurse and family together must create a positive, accepting environment that acts as a stimulus to the establishment and maintenance of effective verbal communication.

The most obvious improvement in the patient's speech will take place within the first six months following the cerebral vascular accident. After that the gains in his ability to communicate will be small and gradual. His relearning to speak will be a long-term process that demands hard work on the part of all concerned—patient, rehabilitation staff, and family. When and if the patient returns home, the family assumes responsibility for encouraging speech. Only a well-informed and understanding family can maintain an environment conducive to speech recovery.

Hemiplegia

Hemiplegia is the paralysis of one side of the body. Initially, the paralysis is flaccid in nature; then it progresses to a rigid or spastic paralysis. It is accompanied by a variety of other problems, including numbness and muscle weakness on the involved side, poor balance, poor muscle control, lack of stamina and easy fatigue, edema of tissues of the affected limbs, and pain in the extremities, especially the shoulder. The patient's perception of himself, his illness, and his environment is greatly affected by the brain injury. His sense of touch and his awareness of movement and position in space on the involved side may be lost. Visual problems increase and compound the perceptual problems. The patient is especially prone to hemianopsia, which is defective vision or blindness in one half of the visual field. Confusion and disorientation frequently occur with left-sided hemiplegia, and aphasia with right-sided paralysis.

In addition to the physical and perceptual problems associated with hemiplegia, the patient will manifest various psychological problems. For seemingly no reason the patient will go from a depressed state to one of extreme elation. These rapid mood swings are described as emotional lability. Loss of memory, shortened attention span, irresponsible and unsafe actions are also concurrent problems. The patient may deny his illness because he cannot comprehend what has happened to him. He is terribly confused; his ability to communicate is diminished or absent (due to scrambled perceptual input and mixed verbal output), and he is afraid that he is going insane.

Throughout the entire rehabilitation program, the patient's most common emotion will be frustration. Every new step he tries to take will be a giant hurdle to cross. Each new effort will increase his frustration. His frustration may be expressed by anger or crying.

Care of the hemiplegic patient who is confined to bed will be based on the nursing principles discussed in Chapter 6, although these principles have to be modified and specific nursing measures applied when the patient has suffered a stroke.

Since the hemiplegic patient cannot control muscular activity in the affected areas, it is vital for him to be properly positioned. Good body alignment must be instituted upon the patient's admission to the hospital. It is especially important for good body alignment to be maintained during the period of flaccid paralysis, when the limbs are limp and easy to position, so that when spasticity occurs, the patient will not acquire a handicap worse than his hemiplegia. Initially, the limbs assume a characteristic position of poor body alignment. The paralyzed leg is in outward rotation; the knee is flexed; and the foot is dropped. The patient's arm is held close to the body, and his elbow, fingers, and thumb are flexed. A trochanter roll (sandbag or rolled heavy pillow) may be placed alongside the hip, or the trochanter, on the affected side to relieve the outward rotation. The feet should be placed firmly against a footboard. The patient should lie flat in bed except to perform activities of daily living. Sitting up in bed for a long period of time could lead to a flexion contracture of the hip. A pillow should be placed between the patient's arm and his chest in order to prevent adduction of the shoulder. His arm, wrist, and elbow should be elevated on a pillow. This position will help to prevent edema in the affected upper extremity. A rolled washcloth or small towel should be used to position the hand, so that the fingers are slightly flexed and the thumb is in opposition to the other digits.

In order to prevent the complications that can arise from enforced immobility, the patient should be turned at least every two hours. At this time he may be placed in the prone position with a small pillow under his pelvis for support. His toes should hang over the end of the mattress. A hand roll is still used to maintain proper positioning of his hand. Any side-lying position may be used as long as the patient lies on his unaffected side. He should never be positioned on his affected side. Skin surfaces should be separated from each other by pillows, and his affected hip should not be sharply flexed. Hands and feet must be properly positioned. (See Figure 10-1.)

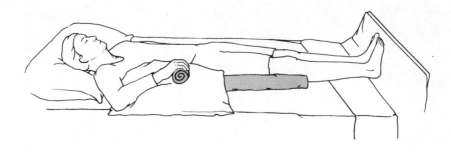

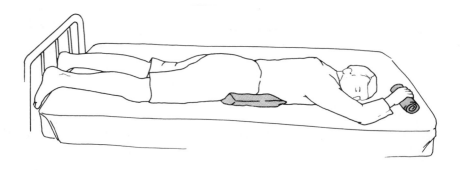

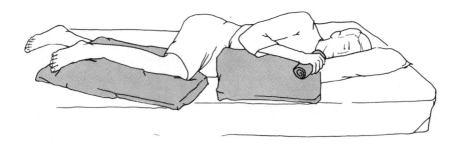

Figure 10-1: Proper positioning of hemiplegic patient. (From top to bottom) Supine, Prone, Side.

Range-of-motion exercises should be performed on all joints. Of special importance are the joints and muscles of the unaffected side of the body, since they will be used for moving, weight bearing, and locomotion. If the patient can understand directions, he may be taught to use his unaffected arm to exercise the hemiplegic side. The range-of-motion exercises will be the same as those discussed in earlier chapters. However, the nurse should bear in mind that the patient may not be able to inform her of any discomfort during the exercises, due to lack of feeling and of aphasia when present. The nurse should move all joints through the range of motion with caution, since any preexisting limitations will be unknown.

The patient's shoulder may become painful due to the force of gravity pulling the paralyzed arm downward and thereby causing an incomplete dislocation of the shoulder. This can be prevented by having the patient use a sling when he is sitting or standing. A pillow support will serve as a preventive measure for the bedfast patient. If a sling is used constantly, the lack of exercise will cause a frozen shoulder. Consequently, the sling must be removed at regular intervals to permit exercise of the shoulder. The physician will order special exercises involving the rope and pulley, and the patient will perform these in the physical therapy department. The sling is usually worn until the affected arm has developed severe spasticity or until there is some evidence of shoulder-shrugging ability.

As soon as the patient's medical condition stabilizes, the physician will allow him out of bed. The wheelchair may need special features, such as a one-arm drive and a special arm support, to meet the needs of the hemiplegic patient.

If the patient has difficulty with comprehension, the nursing team must develop a consistent and exact procedure for transfers, locomotion, and ambulation. Some basic pointers are:

1. Use simple directions and short commands.
2. Repeat instructions often.
3. Demonstrate procedures to the patient—one step at a time.
4. Be patient—give him time to follow directions.
5. Offer praise and encouragement—even for his trying.

The patient's ability to understand and follow verbal instructions should be evaluated. Physical reasons for poor comprehension, such as deafness or vision problems, will have to be corrected with glasses or hearing aids before transfers can be successfully taught. Some patients will have such severe problems with vision (hemianopsia) and spatial relationships that they may never progress to locomotion and ambulation.

Ambulation is preceded by a series of standing activities, such as transfers and exercise. These are carried out in the physical therapy department and practiced and reinforced in the nursing unit when the patient carries out his activities of daily living.

The hemiplegic patient will need special aids to ambulation. A short leg brace will provide support and assist the patient in acquiring balance for walking. The brace will be equipped with a ninety-degree posterior stop, which will prevent plantar flexion, or foot drop. (See Figure 10-3.) An outer T-strap will also be added to prevent inward turning of the foot. Long leg braces are utilized by patients who lack stability of the lower limb.

The hemiplegic patient will need some type of support, either a cane or crutch, for locomotion. The physical therapist will teach the patient the proper gait after the preparatory exercise training. Nurses should know the gait pattern and encourage and support the patient during his locomotion efforts. A typical gait pattern with cane might be:

1. The patient stands with his weight on both feet.
2. The cane is held in his unaffected hand.
3. The cane is advanced.

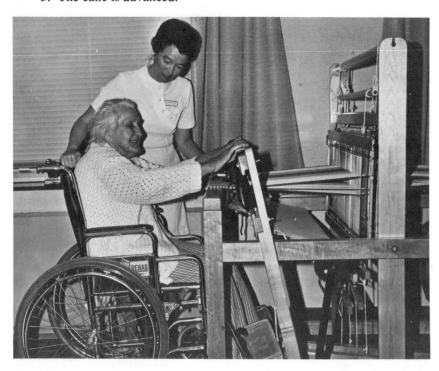

Figure 10-2: Use of the loom strengthens arm and leg muscles. Occupational therapist assists in proper technique.

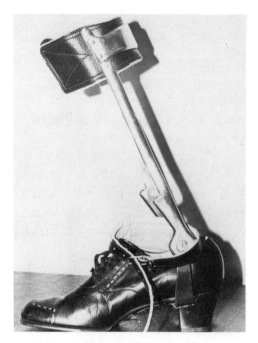

Figure 10-3: Short leg brace for hemiplegic patient.

4. The involved leg is advanced.

5. The normal leg is advanced.

When helping the patient to walk, the nurse should offer support on the affected side, since he is most likely to fall toward this side. The patient should keep the cane fairly close to his body in order to provide a good base of support. Additional activities of locomotion, such as ascending and descending stairs, will be taught in the physical therapy department.

The patient should attempt activities of daily living as early as possible. These activities will help him to reestablish self-care and will serve to strengthen his unaffected limbs. As soon as the patient can sit out of bed for half an hour, he may begin self-feeding, even though the procedure will be difficult. The patient will experience general weakness because of his illness, and he may be forced to use his left hand when he is really right-handed or vice versa. Futhermore, weakened facial muscles, lack of tongue control, and ill-fitting dentures will make chewing difficult. Food may lodge between the teeth and the side of the mouth on the affected side. If there is pronounced muscular weakness on the hemiplegic side of the face, the patient may have difficulty sipping liquids from a glass or cup. The patient's clothing should be protected with a large towel when he is relearning to feed himself. Foods should have a low spill factor and should be relatively easy to cut and chew. Help should be given as necessary. The meal should be arranged to allow for ease in feeding, and only one or two utensils should be provided. The tray should be set for simplicity, not formal elegance. If hemianopsia is present, the patient may not see the entire plate and may not eat all the food. Rotating the plate will help the patient to see the entire meal.

The patient can begin other activities of daily living by assisting with bathing his face and hands. As time passes, he will assume more responsibility for self-care. The patient's ability to care for his own personal hygiene usually increases with locomotion and ambulation. The nurse will need to check the affected hand, axilla, elbow, and groin for proper cleansing and drying. Skin irritation is apt to occur in these areas due to lack of exercise, edema, or incontinence. Tub or shower baths may be instituted when the patient can successfully accomplish this type of transfer. Many aids to daily living are available to help the hemiplegic patient in his program of personal hygiene. Denture brushes, nail brushes, and even cakes of soap can be attached to the inside of the sink by suction cups. Patients will need assistance with some aspects of grooming. Women will need to have their hair shampooed and styled, and men will need to have someone connect their electric razors. Patients with hemianopsia will need to be reminded about grooming the sides of their faces.

Bowel and bladder training will be instituted as soon as the patient is able to participate in such a program. Good results are achieved when he is able to sit up and use the commode for elimination. The general principles for a bowel and bladder training program have already been discussed.

The patient will find dressing with only one side of his body fully functioning a very taxing and frustrating procedure. The nurse can ease the task by using the pointers discussed in earlier chapters. In addition, there are some specific hints that may help the hemiplegic patient. When dressing, he should begin with the involved extremity, using the strong limb to do the work. When he undresses, he should start with his normal limb. Labels on clothing will help the patient to distinguish the front from the back and the inside from the outside. It will be easier for him to dress if he has good sitting balance and can place both feet on the floor. Shoes and socks may be easier to put on if he can put his feet on a footstool to obtain a more convenient working height. Long-handled or regular shoehorns can be used. Putting on a shoe and brace is an even more complicated process and is usually taught in the physical therapy department. The patient's affected arm is put in a sling after he is fully clothed. The sling should be a type that the patient can apply and remove himself, so that he can carry out prescribed exercise to prevent shoulder pain and deformity.

Efforts must be made to prevent the patient from becoming socially isolated. Group dining is an excellent way for patients to reestablish social contact. Group exercises, especially range-of-motion exercises for the affected arm, provide fun with a purpose. Visits from family and friends will lift the patient's spirits and outlook. The telephone, too, can be an instrument of socialization. However, the patient may need reeducation in dialing, answering the telephone and speaking on it. Furthermore, it must be within his reach. Newspapers and magazines will help the patient to keep in touch with the outside world. Aphasia and hemianopsia may interfere with the patient's reading ability, but the nurse should assume that the patient has some understanding of the written word.

Prognosis

An early return of function is considered an encouraging sign. If complete recovery is to occur, it can be expected within two months. Should total recovery not occur, the patient is left with residual hemiplegia, which may be complete or incomplete. However, improvement of function can still occur, particularly if there are no other concurrent disabilities. About 85 percent of all hemiplegic patients can learn to walk and perform self-care activities.

Discharge

Once the patient has achieved his maximum potential, he will be discharged. Planning for the patient's return home will include special provisions. The housewife who has suffered a stroke will have special training in occupational therapy, which will help her to resume home duties. Single men may also require this type of training. Sometimes a visiting homemaker service will be called upon to assist with the management of the home.

Patients with significant residual problems will need expert nursing care in the home, which will be provided by the public health nursing agency in the community. In time the visiting nurse may teach the family to care for the patient. If this is not possible, a home health aide may give routine care to the patient. Supervision and health maintenance visits will be the responsibility of the public health nurse. (See Figure 10-4.)

In some areas of the United States discharged hemiplegic patients meet in stroke clubs. These gatherings help to prevent depression and loss of physical gains at a time when the patient and his family really have to go

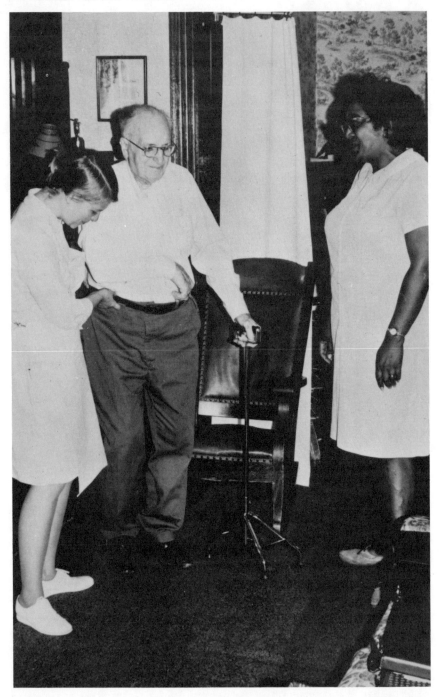

Figure 10-4: Visiting nurse and homemaker observe patient using the quad cane.

it alone. Also these clubs provide the social rehabilitation that might otherwise be lacking, so that the patient is not completely homebound.

Some patients may be so limited in their physical and mental abilities that they will need constant custodial care in a nursing home. Even though these patients have no further potential for improvement, they still require skilled and loving nursing care. Constant vigilance is essential to prevent the complications that occur as a result of immobility and hemiplegia.

Research

Stroke research centers have been established throughout the country. Their purpose is to learn more about causes of strokes and ways in which they can be prevented or controlled. Many physical rehabilitation centers and departments of physical medicine within hospitals have programs of rehabilitation specially designed for the stroke victim in which new rehabilitation techniques are being developed.

EMPHYSEMA

Emphysema is one of several diseases that fall under the category of chronic obstructive pulmonary diseases, (COPD). Asthma and acute and chronic bronchitis are also included in this group. Emphysema is characterized by irreversible changes in the anatomy of the lungs causing the elastic properties of the lungs, particularly of the alveoli, to be reduced. The term comes from the Greek word meaning inflated. In fact, there is a ballooning out, or blistering, of the alveoli, resulting in the destruction of some of the alveolar walls and capillary beds. Because these walls are stretched, their ability to contract and force out the air is reduced, and the lungs remain overinflated with air. As a result, the opportunity for exchange of oxygen and carbon dioxide between the capillaries and alveoli is diminished.

Approximately 10 million Americans have the disease. It is more prevalent in white males, particularly between the ages of fifty and seventy, than in nonwhites or females. Over the past ten years there has been a phenomenal (approximately 800 percent) increase in the disease. Although the cause of the disease is unknown, air pollution has played a definite role in the rapid growth of cases over the years. Other contributing factors are heavy cigarette smoking and conditions that result in severe scarring of the lungs, such as silicosis and chronic bronchitis.

The onset of the disease is so gradual that the patient is usually not able to give a clear picture of the beginning of his symptoms. A detailed medical history will reveal evidence of a persistent cough, usually producing mucous sputum, and a series of upper respiratory infections particularly during the winter months. The symptom that usually brings the patient to the physician is increasing episodes of dyspnea. At first, the patient may attribute dyspnea upon exertion to his growing old. Unfortunately, this is not the case, and eventually it becomes difficult for him to breathe even without physical activity.

As these irreversible respiratory changes take place, the patient is forced to use all his energies in an effort to breathe. Accessory muscles of respiration, such as the muscles of the neck and shoulders, are brought into play in an effort to raise the thorax. Neck veins also become more prominent. Inhaling is not as difficult as exhaling. The emphysema victim may purse his lips in an attempt to provide the pressure needed to force out the air trapped in his lungs. Exhalation will be prolonged. As the disease progresses, it becomes harder for the patient to breathe, and more air is trapped in the lungs. In some cases the rib cage enlarges into a characteristic barrel chest. In turn, the diaphragm flattens, hardly moving during exhalation. Through experimentation the patient usually finds that dyspnea is lessened if he sits bent forward in a chair. This position allows greater room for the diaphragm to expand and contract. Some patients will find that this bent-forward stance is also helpful when they are standing and walking.

As dyspnea increases, cyanosis of the lips, nail beds, and skin will be noticed. Exhalation becomes more forced, causing the pressure within the thoracic cavity to increase. Eventually the pressure causes a narrowing of the bronchi and bronchioles. As stated previously, susceptibility to upper respiratory infections increases. Infectious organisms cause edema of the mucous membrane linings throughout the lung, contributing to further narrowing. The patient has increasing difficulty trying to remove secretions by coughing. Thus, mucous secretions are retained, become thickened, and are more difficult to expel. Most of these patients are mouth breathers, which further contributes to a drying out of secretions and the creation of hard, thick plugs of mucus.

Because the circulatory and respiratory systems are so totally dependent on each other, advanced emphysema will have a profound effect on the functioning of the circulatory system. A large percentage of the capillary beds that come in contact with the alveoli are destroyed, and the backup of blood in the pulmonary artery causes pressure to increase, which leads to increased pressure within the right ventricle of the heart. In fact, the entire heart becomes overworked in an effort to handle the situation, which results in the condition called cor pulmonale. This is a secondary heart disease resulting from the heart's unsuccessful effort to compensate for the blockage caused by obstruction in the lungs. Most emphysematous patients succumb to heart failure.

Diagnosis of emphysema is made through careful physical examination and fluoroscopy. Lateral chest X rays may also be ordered, since they will show evidence of the flattened diaphragm and the depth of the chest. The routine flat chest X ray will not show changes due to emphysema. Accurate, careful, history taking by the physician is important. A test of the patient's vital lung capacity will be ordered. This test measures the amount of air the patient can forcefully exhale following the deepest breath he can take. A meter records the amount of exhaled gas. In patients who have had emphysema for some time, the complete blood count will reveal an increase in red blood cells. This phenomenon is the body's attempt to increase the oxygen-carrying capability of the blood.

Since neither the cause nor a cure for emphysema has yet been found, treatment and rehabilitation are geared to delaying further progression of the disease and to relieving respiratory obstruction. Patients are also assisted in utilizing their maximum ability to function. Both the patient and his family must learn to live within the limits of the patient's disability and to adapt their style of living to accommodate an appropriate therapy regimen. Although the patient is confined to a hospital for treatment of an acute respiratory crisis, most of the time he is usually in his own home. Care in a nursing home or rehabilitation center may be indicated, but only for short durations.

Delaying Further Progression

One of the constant threats to the emphysematous patient is upper respiratory infection. Some physicians will order antibiotics as a prophylactic measure. Others will order medication only when there is evidence that the patient has been exposed to these infections. The patient and his family need to be extra cautious in preventing respiratory infections.

Since one of the problems associated with emphysema is constriction of the bronchial tree, bronchodilatory drugs may be ordered. These drugs serve as a means of relieving constriction, allowing oxygen to get to more alveoli, and allowing mucus to be cleared more easily. They may be given orally, subcutaneously, or by nebulization. When taking the drug by nebulization, the patient administers it directly into the bronchial tree by inhaling an aerosol mist of medication. Small portable nebulizers, which can be carried in the patient's pocket, emit measured dosages of medication in each spray (metered mist). Immediate improvement in breathing results, but effects are brief. Aminophylline rectal suppositories may also be effective.

Bronchodilators may also be administered by means of the intermittent positive pressure breathing (IPPB) apparatus. This machine assists the patient in ventilating those areas of the lung that have had poor aeration. The patient breathes pressurized air or oxygen with medication. Slow, even respirations, proper posture, and physical relaxation are essential if maximum effects are to be achieved. The physician will order the amount of treatment with IPPB. Because IPPB treatments do increase the patient's functioning capacities in some cases, the physician may prescribe the machine's regular use. An inhalation therapist can give these treatments on an outpatient basis in a hospital clinic or in his office. The patient may prefer to purchase the machine for use at home if the physician so prescribes.

The physician may order other drugs to help liquefy thick mucous secretions and ease expectoration. There are times when the patient may require oxygen therapy. For example, when an upper respiratory infection limits the already diminished capacity to breathe, hypoxia exists, and there is a need for prolonged use of oxygen. The patient will be admitted to the hospital or nursing home so that the proper oxygen therapy can be administered. Oxygen may be delivered to the patient by nasal catheter or cannula or by a face mask or tent, the face mask being the most effective means of increasing the percentage of inhaled oxygen.

Utilizing the Patient's Maximum Ability to Function

If one of the factors contributing to emphysema is a polluted environment, it is reasonable to conclude that an environment with relatively clean air will be helpful to the patient. One of the first orders given to the emphysema victim who smokes is to stop smoking immediately. Family members who smoke should also be encouraged to quit or to avoid smoking in the patient's presence. Other airborne irritants, such as dust, fumes, and smog, should be reduced to a minimum. The patient and his family need to know practical ways of avoiding or reducing these irritating substances.

Since the patient uses a great deal of energy in the process of breathing, it is understandable that his energy reserves will be depleted quickly. A part of the rehabilitation process is to help the patient increase his activity tolerance and decrease the energy expended solely on breathing. A program of increased exercises may be ordered. The patient will find the time immediately after he arises in the morning particularly difficult. Bronchial secretions accumulated during the night must be raised, and coughing up thickened mucous plugs is usually very exhausting. If the nurse gives the patient a hot drink when he arises, it will help to liquefy the material.

Perhaps the greatest assistance the nurse can give during this trying period is to let the routine morning care activities wait till later in the day. Calm, supportive reassurance can help the patient greatly in getting over the difficult morning.

Anxiety-producing situations should be avoided, since they lead to further difficulties in breathing. Rushing the patient to finish his bath or meal or hurrying him off for treatment reduces the ultimate effectiveness of all therapy. Preparation for trips to physical therapy and other departments in the hospital, nursing home, or rehabilitation center should be made well in advance, so that pressures on the patient are reduced to a minimum. In addition to the time following morning rising, there will be other periods, such as the time following the evening meal, when the patient's activity tolerance is particularly low. Rest should be encouraged and activity requirements reduced during these times.

The patient's diet should include adequate fluids, especially water, which helps to liquefy secretions. Gas-forming foods should be eliminated from the diet, since they may cause interference with abdominal breathing. If the patient is given frequent small feedings rather than three large meals per day, his fatigue will be reduced and his energy conserved.

One of the major changes in the life of the emphysema patient will be his method of breathing. The physician may order respiratory exercises, which the physical therapist will teach the patient. Through abdominal breathing exercises the patient will learn to use muscles of the abdomen and chest in order to breathe properly. Controlled, slow respirations with emphasis on emptying the lungs as completely as possible will be practiced with the therapist assisting the patient. Exercises will also help the patient to relax. The physical therapist may also teach the patient postural drainage techniques along with other respiratory exercises. Proper coughing technique and posture will also be explained. The nurse will assist the patient in carrying out his exercises in the patient care unit. She needs to report any problems the patient has with his exercises to the therapist. The nurse should be on the lookout for signs of the patient's reverting to short, quick respirations and mouth breathing rather than following the directions given to him for proper respiratory exercises. Encouragement must be given to the emphysema victim so that he will persevere in these most essential exercises.

Living Within the Limits of Disability

We all have experienced moments when we couldn't catch our breath, and we know what a frightening feeling it can be. The emphysema patient learns to live with this fear on a day-to-day basis, and his family also must adapt to this fear. The act of breathing, which was once an automatic function, now becomes a conscious effort with each respiration. Panic on the part of both the patient and his family during coughing episodes can lead to more anxiety; all are waiting for the next bout to occur. The patient's fear of dying is very real and results in periods of depression. If the family and patient understand the disease and know how to cope with its symptoms, fear, panic, and anxiety can be greatly reduced. Depression can be replaced with hope, but only with continuous positive efforts on the part of all members of the family. Emphysema clubs for patients and their families have been formed in various communities. Expert help in dealing with the problems arising from this disease and psychological support are given to the members of these clubs.

Perhaps one of the first things to cross the patient's mind is the thought of moving to a warmer, drier climate in order to cope with the problem. Although the incidence of upper respiratory infections is not as great in warm, dry areas as in damp, cold climates, not all emphysema patients react favorably to a change in environment. Before making a permanent change in residence, the patient and family should visit the proposed new location for several months. In this way the patient can determine whether, in fact, any benefit would be derived from a permanent change. A two-week trip may provide temporary relief of symptoms, but this relief may prove to be misleading in the long run.

The patient living at home should avoid exposure to very cold air, since the bronchial tree will react by further constriction. If the patient lives alone perhaps he can make arrangements with neighbors to run errands when necessary during hazardous weather. If a meal on wheels program is available in the community, it should be utilized by the emphysema patient. If the patient must go out of doors during very cold weather, he should wear a scarf over his nose and mouth. Conversely, during very warm, humid weather at least one room in the house should be equipped with an air conditioner to provide relief.

The public health nurse may assist the patient and his family in setting up a realistic plan of daily activities that incorporates those therapies that have already been discussed. Because the first few hours after the patient arises usually present specific difficulties, a routine may need to be devised that will help both the patient and his family at this time.

An established daily routine not only provides the components necessary for an effective therapeutic regimen but also helps the patient and his family to concentrate on the positive, active benefits that can be derived from this regimen.

STUDY QUESTIONS AND PROBLEMS

1. Mr. Michaels suffered a cerebral vascular accident approximately six weeks ago. He has shown no progress in resuming activities of daily living, locomotion, or ambulation. He has right hemiplegia, does not speak or communicate, is completely withdrawn, has no interest in his environment, and is incontinent of urine and feces. He has been admitted to a nursing home for custodial care, since he is not expected to benefit from any program of rehabilitation. Prepare a nursing care plan to meet Mr. Michaels' needs and to prevent the problems that can arise during prolonged immobilization.

2. Mrs. Jervis, who has also had a cerebral vascular accident, has been in a rehabilitation center for three weeks. She is progressing in her program of rehabilitation and is beginning to walk with the aid of the walker. She has learned to apply her brace, and perform almost all activities of daily living by herself.

   Her major difficulty is with her speech. She has expressive aphasia and will not talk because she makes so many errors. She feels she should progress with speech therapy as readily as with physical and occupational therapy. Mrs. Jervis' children are deeply concerned about their mother's aphasia and apparent lack of progress. They are aware of the high expectations she has always set for herself.

   How can the nurse help Mrs. Jervis and her family to understand the progress of speech therapy? What can the family and the nurse do to encourage Mrs. Jervis to attempt verbal communication?

BIBLIOGRAPHY

Agranowitz, Aleen, and McKeown, Milfred. *Aphasia Handbook for Adults and Children.* Springfield, Ill.: Charles C. Thomas, 1964.

Ballantyne, Donna. "Evaluating ADL at the Bedside." *American Journal of Nursing,* November 1966, pp. 2440–2441.

Barach, Alvan L. *A Treatment Manual for Patients with Pulmonary Emphysema.* New York: Grune & Stratton, 1969.

Beeson, Paul, and McDermott, Walsh, eds. *Textbook of Medicine.* 12th ed. Philadelphia: W. B. Saunders, 1967.

Brunner, Lillian; Emerson, Charles; Ferguson, Kraeer; and Suddath, Doris. *Textbook of Medical-Surgical Nursing.* 2nd ed. Philadelphia: J. B. Lippincott, 1970.

Buck, McKenzie. *Dysphasia—Professional Guidance for Family and Patient.* Englewood Cliffs, N.J.: Prentice-Hall, 1968.

Burt, Margaret M. "Perceptual Deficits in Hemiplegia." *American Journal of Nursing,* May 1970, pp. 1026–1029.

Chronic Obstructive Pulmonary Disease. New York: National Tuberculosis and Respiratory Disease Association, 1972.

Departments of Occupational Therapy and Nursing Education at Kenny Rehabilitation Institute. *Self-Care for the Hemiplegic.* Minneapolis: American Rehabilitation Foundation, 1970.

Flaherty, Patricia Toohey, and Jurkovich, Sandra J. *Transfers for Patients with Acute and Chronic Conditions.* Minneapolis: American Rehabilitation Foundation, 1970.

Gerdes, Lenore. "The Confused or Delirious Patient." *American Journal of Nursing,* June 1968, p. 1229.

Griffin, Winnie; Anderson, Sara J.; and Pasor, Joyce Y. "Group Exercise for Patients with Limited Motion." *American Journal of Nursing,* September 1971, pp. 1742–1743.

Helming, Mary G., ed. *Nursing in Respiratory Diseases, A Symposium.* Nursing Clinics of North America, September, 1968.

Hirschberg, Gerald G.; Lewis, Leon; and Thomas, Dorothy. *Rehabilitation: A Manual for the Care of the Disabled and Elderly.* Philadelphia: J. B. Lippincott, 1964.

Introduction to Respiratory Diseases. 4th ed. New York: National Tuberculosis and Respiratory Disease Association, 1969.

Lowman, Edward, and Klinger, Judith L. *Aids to Independent Living.* New York: McGraw-Hill, 1969.

Martin, Nancy; King, Rosemarie; and Suchinski, Joyce. "The Nurse Therapist in a Rehabilitation Setting." *American Journal of Nursing,* August 1970, pp. 1694–1697.

Miller, Barbara E. "Assisting Aphasic Patients with Speech Rehabilitation." *American Journal of Nursing,* May 1969.

Nett, Louise M., and Petty, Thomas L. "Why Emphysema Patients Are the Way They Are." *American Journal of Nursing,* June 1970.

Obley, Fred A. *Emphysema—A Doctor's Advice for Patients and Their Families.* Boston: Beacon Press, 1970.

Piskar, Barbara K., and Paleos, Sonia. "The Group Way to Banish After Stroke Blues." *American Journal of Nursing,* July 1968, p. 1500.

Robley, Spencer H. *Emphysema and Common Sense.* West Nyack, N.Y.: Parker Publishing Company, 1968.

Rossman, Isadore. *Clinical Geriatrics.* Philadelphia: J. B. Lippincott, 1968.

Sarno, John E., and Sarno, Martha Taylor. *Stroke—The Condition and the Patient.* New York: McGraw-Hill, 1969.

Schuell, Hildred; Jenkins, James J.; and Jimenez-Pabon, Edward. *Aphasia in Adults.* New York: Harper & Row, 1964.

Schwaid, Madeline C. "The Impact of Emphysema." *American Journal of Nursing,* June 1970.

Smith, Dorothy; Germain, Carol; and Gips, Claudia. *Care of the Adult Patient.* 3rd ed. Philadelphia: J. B. Lippincott, 1971.

Sorenson, Lois, and Ulrich, Patricia. *Ambulation: A Manual for Nurses.* Rehabilitation Publication, no. 707. Minneapolis: American Rehabilitation Institute, 1966.

Strike Back at Stroke. New York: American Heart Association, 1967.

Up and Around—A Booklet to Aid the Stroke Patient in Activities of Daily Living. New York: American Heart Association, 1967.

What You Can Do About Your Breathing. New York: National Tuberculosis Association, 1967.

Wolcott, Lester, and Wheeler, Paul. "Rehabilitation and the Aged," in U.S., Department of Health, Education, and Welfare, *Working with Older People—A Guide to Practice,* vol. 4, *Clinical Aspects of Aging,* Austin B. Chinn, ed. Washington, D.C.: U.S. Government Printing Office, 1971.

11

Restorative Nursing of Patients with Diabetes Mellitus

Diabetes mellitus is a condition characterized by hyperglycemia or a chronic increase in blood sugar. This excess is caused by an absence or insufficient production of insulin. Insulin is manufactured in the islets of Langerhans, special groups of cells located in the pancreas, and sent directly into the blood stream. The hormone is essential in the utilization and storage of the sugar that the body has derived from food, and when it is absent or in short supply, sugar begins to accumulate in the bloodstream. The body makes several attempts to correct this condition. When hyperglycemia reaches a certain level, the sugar is spilled over from the kidneys into the urine. Thus, there are two primary symptoms of diabetes: polyuria, or frequent urination, and glycosuria, or sugar in the urine. Since the kidneys excrete large amounts of fluids, the patient is very thirsty and drinks huge quantities, a condition known as polydipsia. Although the glucose in the bloodstream is more than plentiful, it cannot be utilized by the body due to the lack of insulin. Therefore, the patient will have an increased appetite (polyphagia) and a loss in weight. Since the body cannot utilize glucose for energy, fats and proteins are used for this purpose. Normally, these substances are stored or deposited in the body cells. Ketone bodies (acid substances) are a by-product of the incomplete metabolism of fats. One of these ketone bodies is acetone. When these substances accumulate in the blood, a condition known as diabetic acidosis develops.

INCIDENCE

There are approximately 2 million diagnosed diabetics in the United States, and it is estimated that another 2 million are undiagnosed. Furthermore, it is estimated that there are 5 million potential diabetics in the present population. The incidence of this disease increases as age increases. In fact, 85 percent of all diabetics are over forty-five, and some 40 percent are over sixty-five. Some researchers have reported that the elderly have a decreased ability to utilize glucose. Whether this is a normal part of the aging process or mild or predisposing diabetes is not known. Those who are most prone to the disease include women who have a history of having large babies (nine pounds or over) or an unusual obstetric history (recurrent abortions, toxemias, stillbirths, etc.), those with a family history of diabetes, and those who are obese.

SYMPTOMS

The classic symptoms of diabetes are polyuria, polyphagia, polydipsia, and glycosuria, accompanied by a feeling of fatigue and weight loss. These symptoms are found in the individual who develops juvenile diabetes. This form of the disease usually occurs during youth, although it has been known to develop during maturity. The juvenile diabetic lacks insulin in his body and is dependent on injections of this hormone, which is the basis of his treatment. When diabetes develops later in life, the patient usually has some ability to produce insulin and may be treated with the oral hypoglycemic drugs. Most often the mature patient goes to the doctor because of a complication of the undiagnosed disease. A few of the many observations that might lead the physician to suspect diabetes and investigate further are eye problems (such as cataracts, glaucoma, and retinal changes), severe itching, infections, leg and foot ulcers leading to gangrene, and coronary artery disease.

DIAGNOSIS

When the laboratory findings show hyperglycemia and glycosuria, they indicate the need for more specific diagnostic studies. The physician will usually order a two-hour postprandial blood sugar test. The most meaningful test is the standard glucose tolerance test. For at least three days prior to the test, the patient is given a diet that is very high in carbohydrates. On the day of the test a fasting blood sugar is drawn. Following this the patient is administered a standard dose of glucose orally. Blood samples are taken for glucose content at half-hour intervals for at least three hours. There are many highly specialized laboratory tests that the doctor may order to further pinpoint the diagnosis.

TREATMENT

One of the basics of treatment is the prescription of a diet that will provide satisfactory nutrition, meet energy requirements, attain or maintain
normal weight, and prevent hyperglycemia and glycosuria. In some elderly
diabetics dietary modification may be all that is necessary to control the
disease process. Most physicians, however, do not impose rigid dietary
regulations on elderly patients. Such an approach is most frightening to
the patient, and he may become anxious, confused, and depressed. This
does not mean that the patient can eat anything he likes. His diet must be
nutritionally sound and provide adequate calories for his age and exercise
level. Proteins must be of high quality and in sufficient quantity to maintain the life-supporting systems. Carbohydrate intake is usually restricted,
but the diet must be carefully balanced to allow for proper fat and protein
metabolism. Patients are instructed to avoid simple sugars and highly re-
fined carbohydrates. The chief sources of carbohydrate intake should be
cereal, breads, vegetables, and fruits, which are complex sugars and consequently will be absorbed and metabolized slowly. Certainly, sugar, honey,
syrups, pies, cakes, donuts, etc., are prohibited. Fats are usually limited in
quantity, because they are the most concentrated form of energy. Some
doctors recommend that the patient obtain his fat intake from polyunsatu-
rated fats in order to lower the blood cholesterol level and thus reduce
the likelihood of coronary artery disease. Whether or not a diet low in
polyunsaturates is indeed effective in disease prevention remains a matter
of much discussion among researchers and physicians.

When dietary treatment does not control the disease process sufficiently, the doctor will order one of the oral hypoglycemic drugs. These
are used primarily by the patient whose diabetes develops in the mature
years. These drugs fall into two broad categories: the sulfonylureas and
phenformin. The sulfonylurea drugs, such as Orinase and Diabinese cause
insulin to be secreted by the beta cells in the islets of Langerhans. Phenformin, known as DBI, appears to supplement the insulin that is already
present in the body. The dosage of these drugs will vary for each patient
and may have to be altered periodically to meet his needs. Further information on the oral hypoglycemics may be found in a current pharmacology
text. At the time of this writing the oral hypoglycemics are under intensive
investigation by the United States Food and Drug Administration. Some
researchers feel that complications may arise from these drugs, and the un-
desirable effects may be more severe than the diabetes itself. Therefore, the
reader is encouraged to consult current literature on these drugs in order to
determine their present status.

Insulin is not used regularly by the elderly diabetic, but rather is utilized only when the patient has demonstrated a clinical need for the hormone. Acute problems such as ketosis, failure to respond to the oral drugs, and the persistence of the symptoms of diabetes would indicate a need for insulin. Therefore, regular insulin may be prescribed in small doses. Usually, the patient responds very well. Some elderly patients may require insulin with a longer lasting effect than regular insulin. The nurse should know the kind of insulin the patient is taking, as well as the times when the hormone begins its action, when it reaches its peak, and when the effectiveness diminishes.

HYPOGLYCEMIA

Lowered blood sugar, or hypoglycemia (insulin reaction) is a severe complication of insulin therapy and of treatment with oral hypoglycemic drugs. Although it occurs infrequently in the elderly diabetic, hypoglycemia may occur swiftly and severely, and it can be fatal for the aged diabetic. The classic symptoms of tachycardia, sweating, and nervousness are generally not experienced by the elderly diabetic patient. Instead, he may become unconscious without any forewarning symptoms. Bizarre or unusual behavior, indicative of hypoglycemia, is easily mistaken for a sign of organic brain damage. The nurse or family needs to be especially vigilant at night, lest the hypoglycemia go unnoticed. Symptoms indicating this state would be nightmares, restlessness, and the inability to be awakened. If the patient can be aroused, the nurse or family should give him orange juice to drink, and the doctor should be notified immediately. When the patient cannot be awakened, glucose will have to be given intravenously. This must be ordered and administered by the physician. If the patient is at home, he should be taken to the emergency room at the local hospital for immediate treatment.

RESTORATIVE NURSING

The main objective of restorative nursing is to help the patient learn more about his condition, adapt his life-style to the requirements necessary to control diabetes, and accept this chronic, irreversible disease. This is a big order. The physician will prescribe the treatment needed; the nurse will help as indicated; but it is the patient who will control the therapy at home. Success or failure in following through the therapy regimen rests squarely with the patient. Therefore, educating him to assume this important role is a serious responsibility for both the physician and the nurse. It is recommended that a reliable family member be present during patient learning sessions, since he or she may be called upon later to perform certain tasks if the patient is unable to do so. These informal sessions are of varying duration and may initially take place in the hospital, the nursing home, or the patient's home. The patient must learn what diabetes is and how it affects the functioning of the body, how to administer insulin or oral hypoglycemics, and how to test the urine. He must also learn the dietary requirements and the signs and symptoms that require immediate treatment and/or medical attention. The importance of maintaining good health and preventing illness must be understood.

Books such as Rosenthal's *Diabetic Care in Pictures* and pamphlets provided by the American Diabetic Association will help the patient to learn. In addition to individualized instruction, the patient may also benefit from group sessions if they are available at the hospital or in the community. The nursing care plan should indicate what progress is being made in the educational process, so that continuity of instruction can be maintained.

The thought of injecting himself with a needle can be frightening to the patient, particularly the elderly patient. The nurse's calm, reassuring, and unhurried approach to this aspect of the patient's education is of vital importance. In addition to instructing the patient on the proper technique for subcutaneous injection, the nurse must stress the importance of giving the prescribed amount of insulin at the same time each day. If the patient skips the medication one day because he feels good or "adds just a wee bit" of insulin because he had a bad day yesterday, he is playing with a lethal weapon. The patient and his family will need to know what equipment is necessary to sterilize the needle and syringe, where to store the material when it is not in use, the technique for sterilizing the equipment, and how to prevent contamination. They must be taught how to attach the needle to the syringe and how to withdraw the insulin from the multidose bottle. When it comes to learning the technique of administering the insulin, the patient can first practice injecting water into an orange to obtain a comparable feel of skin resistance when the needle is inserted into the tissue. In order to assist the patient in selecting sites for insulin injection, the nurse can devise a chart showing the rotation of appropriate locations. (See Figure 11-1.) For patients who have poor eyesight or are partially blind, specially constructed syringes with easier to read markings may be purchased. Adhesive tape markings indicating the level of the correct dosage may help if a standard insulin syringe is used. For the totally blind patient a Cornwall or Tru-Set syringe may be purchased. In this type of syringe the plunger is preset to the correct dosage, so that when it is pulled back, it cannot go beyond this point. A sighted person will need to check the syringe from time to time to make certain it is functioning properly. The importance of keeping an extra syringe and needles on hand, stored in a safe place, should also be stressed. And, of course, the patient should keep enough insulin on hand and should have a set storage space in the refrigerator for this.

Some patients will learn very quickly to administer the insulin injections, because of high motivation and good manual dexterity. When one or both of these factors is poor, it will take the patient longer. In some cases the patient may never acquire the skill, and a family member or public health nurse may have to assume this responsibility. If the patient is at home and has learned to administer his own injections, the public health nurse will visit periodically to check his progress and to reinforce the instructional program. (See Figure 11-2.) If the patient does not require insulin injections, but is placed on oral hypoglycemics, this is considerably easier for him to handle. However, the patient must be instructed to take the medication at the same time each day. The forgetful diabetic should form the habit of taking the pill with the morning meal.

The patient must also be taught the technique of testing the urine for glucose and acetone. Test tape or reagent tablets may be used. For specific instructions concerning urine testing, refer to a standard medical-surgical nursing textbook. The doctor will indicate how frequently the urine should be tested per day and what adjustment in insulin dosage should be made for positive readings. Consequently, the diabetic will need to know the meaning of the color reactions and how to adjust the insulin units.

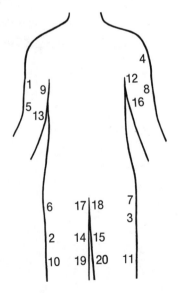

Figure 11-1: One system of rotating injection sites over a 20-day period. A diagram such as this will help the patient to remember the rotation pattern.

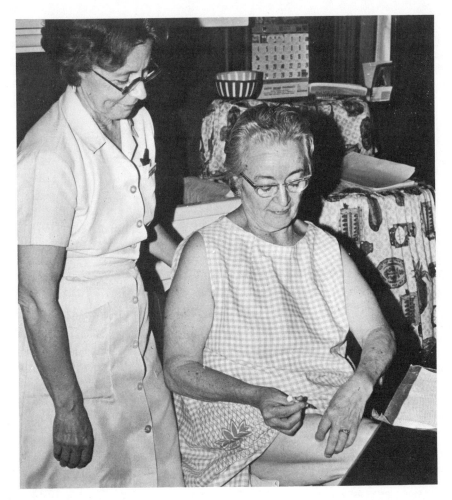

Figure 11-2: Under guidance of the visiting nurse, the patient prepares to inject the insulin.

If reagent tablets are used, they must be stored in a safe, dry place and properly labeled along with the rest of the apparatus for urine testing. A daily record of the tests and their results needs to be kept. The doctor will usually want to review this record periodically.

As has been stated previously, many elderly persons tend to consume high quantities of carbohydrates. The newly diagnosed older diabetic must try to modify such eating patterns, even though they have been well established over the years. This is not an easy task, and some patients may never fully accomplish it, due to their ethnic backgrounds as well as economic factors. A vast majority of persons who eat excessive carbohydrates are overweight, and restrictions on both the amount and the kind of food they are permitted may seem like more than they can bear. The dietitian will instruct the patient and his family concerning the prescribed diet. Perhaps the patient can utilize a diabetic exchange diet as one means of planning appropriate menus. Special emphasis is placed on the patient's setting a given time for meals and adhering to the schedule. In-between meal snacks, particularly at bedtime, may be ordered as part of the total dietary intake per day. These snacks should not be considered extras in addition to what has been prescribed. The drastic consequences of skipping one meal and then doubling up on food intake at the next must be discussed and clearly understood by the patient. The use of expensive dietetic or diabetic products also needs clarification. The physician needs to be consulted regarding the use of these items. The term "dietetic" does not automatically mean free of sugar and can be most misleading. Although the product is usually low in calories, the patient must read the label carefully to determine whether or not sugar content is absent or reduced. For those on limited, fixed incomes, the luxury of diabetic or dietetic foods may not be worth the cost. If a diabetic exchange diet is properly used, it will allow for that helping of ice cream on a special occasion. A review of exchange diets may be found in basic nutrition texts.

The maintenance of health and measures that will help in preventing illness must also be discussed with the older diabetic. He needs to be knowledgeable about the signs and symptoms of infection and realize how essential it is to report these signs immediately to the physician. He should be particularly aware of the signs of upper respiratory infections and of evidence of skin breakdown, especially of lower extremities. Because of the circulatory problems associated with aging and the slow healing process of the diabetic, the importance of meticulous foot care cannot be over-emphasized. This aspect of personal hygiene is often neglected by elderly persons, since poor eyesight and circulatory problems causing dizziness or difficulty in bending down make it difficult to attend to proper foot care. The nurse must emphasize that the patient should carefully wash and dry his feet. Toenails should be filed or, if necessary, cut straight across. For those who have poor eyesight, the toenails should be cut by a family member or chiropodist. For those who can afford periodic visits to a podiatrist or chiropodist, it is money well spent. Many community hospitals have foot clinics as a part of the total diabetic clinic. The patient should also be instructed in the need for properly fitted footwear, which will prevent rubbing and its consequence—skin breakdown.

The patient should also be told of the complications resulting from diabetes. The incidence of cataracts and glaucoma among diabetics is considerable. Signs of peripheral neuritis such as numbness, tingling, and itching, particularly of the legs, need to be reported to the physician.

The importance of follow-up visits to the physician must be stressed and logical reasons given for them. Elderly diabetics often see the trip to the doctor as a luxury they can well do without unless they are "really sick." They must be helped to see that by these routine visits, illness can be prevented and complications discovered before serious results occur. This principle of health teaching is vitally important.

DIABETIC ACIDOSIS

As has been stated, diabetic acidosis occurs when ketone bodies, resulting from the incomplete metabolism of fats, accumulate in the blood. This develops because the body is unable to utilize or store food nutrients. Diabetic acidosis occurs in the diagnosed diabetic when the body's demand for insulin is not met. Various situations can cause this problem. The elderly patient may forget his insulin injection or oral hypoglycemic or feel that he doesn't need it today. He may give himself the injection but miscalculate the dosage and not give himself enough. His body may for some reason need more than the prescribed dosage. (The presence of infections will increase the need for insulin, since the metabolic rate is increased.) He may cheat on his diet, thereby throwing off the delicate balance of the diet and insulin. In all these situations one factor is present— there is not enough insulin to assist the body in metabolizing carbohydrates, proteins, and fats. The diabetes is no longer controlled.

Both patient and family must know the signs and symptoms of diabetic acidosis and the serious consequences if it is left untreated. The course of *untreated* acidosis may be gradual or rapid, leading to coma and death. It may develop slowly over a period of days or weeks. Signs and symptoms include drowsiness and dry, flushed skin. The patient may complain of being thirsty and may have abdominal pain accompanied by vomiting. He becomes dehydrated, which causes the proper balance of body salts to be thrown off. Since the body gets rid of the ketone bodies through the urinary and respiratory systems, a fruity odor may be present in the breath, and acetone will be found in the urine. If the condition is left unchecked, the patient's respirations will become deep and slow (Kussmaul respiration), and his pulse rate will increase. The brain loses its ability to function efficiently, and coma ensues.

Treatment includes restoring the delicate balance of metabolism and electrolytes (body salts), replacing lost fluids, administering proper amounts of insulin, and eventually regulating the diabetic condition. This is a complex procedure, and the patient should be hospitalized immediately. Time is a precious commodity. For this reason all diabetics should carry an identification card similar to that shown in Figure 11-3 or wear a bracelet or medallion.

CONTINUING CARE

Since the major part of the diabetic's life is usually spent at home, continuing supervision may need to be provided by the public health nurse. The nurse should counsel the patient and his family concerning the day-

If unconscious or acting strangely I may be having a reaction to insulin or to an oral medicine taken for diabetes.

I HAVE DIABETES

If I can swallow give me sugar, candy, fruit juice or a sweetened drink. If this does not bring recovery or I can not swallow call a physician or send me to a hospital quickly for administration of glucose or glucagon.

Distributed by
AMERICAN DIABETES ASSOCIATION, INC. • 18 East 48th St. • New York, N.Y. 10017

NAME _____ PHONE _____

ADDRESS _____
(Street) (City) (State)
PHYSICIAN _____ PHONE _____

ADDRESS _____
(Street) (City) (State)

INSULIN	DOSAGE	TIME	ORAL MEDICATION	DOSAGE	TIME
Regular			Orinase		
PZI			Diabinese		
Globin			Dymelor		
NPH			Tolinase		
Lente			DBI		
Semilente			DBI-TD		
Ultralente					

DATE _____ © 1966

Figure 11-3: A sample identification card carried by diabetics.

to-day routines and make sure that the therapy regimen is being carried out properly. Diet counseling by qualified dietitians may be provided through local health departments.

The success of the educational program will depend in large part on the way the patient views himself and his disease. He may react by denying it. He may be uninterested and bored with any instructions. Conversely, he may become so involved in learning and planning his daily routine of care that his world revolves around his illness. Obviously, these are two extremes. Neither is healthy from an emotional point of view. Physician, nurse, patient, and family need to work together, so that the disease aspect is put in the proper perspective. Although there are certain routines that have to be performed to keep the diabetes under control, these routines should not control the elderly diabetic to the exclusion of a meaningful social and healthy emotional life.

STUDY QUESTIONS AND PROBLEMS

1. Mr. and Mrs. McManus were delighted to see the new poster on the bulletin board of the senior citizens' club. A free diabetic-screening clinic would be conducted at the club during the next week. The McManuses know how hard it is to live on a low fixed income, and they really appreciate the value of free health service.

   However, the couple was quite surprised and shocked to find out that they did have high blood sugar. Their doctor prescribed a special diet for both of them and told them to return to his office in two weeks for another blood sugar test. The physician will then determine the need for oral hypoglycemics.

   Obtain samples of the exchange list for diabetic meal planning from the hospital dietitian, your teacher, or a nutrition text, and through role playing, assist Mrs. McManus in working with the exchanges.

2. By the time Mr. Linton got to the diabetic clinic to see about the sore on his toe, it was already gangrenous. This sixty-eight-year-old retired steam fitter was alert, active, and very busy with volunteer activities before he developed diabetes.

   When the ulcerated, gangrenous area failed to respond to medical treatment, the physician recommended a below-the-knee amputation. Mr. Linton agreed to the procedure, and the surgery was performed.

   When the wound had begun to heal, the surgeon allowed Mr. Linton to be out of bed in a wheelchair. Soon he will be transferred to the rehabilitation center for active therapy before ambulation with a prosthesis. The nurses have several goals they wish to accomplish before he leaves the general hospital. How can the nursing personnel help to achieve the following?
   a. Strengthen Mr. Linton's arms in preparation for ambulation
   b. Prevent contracture deformities
   c. Teach transfer to the wheelchair
   d. Review the testing of urine for sugar and acetone
   e. Help Mr. Linton to reestablish an acceptable self-image

BIBLIOGRAPHY

Anderson, Helen C. *Newton's Geriatric Nursing.* 5th ed. Saint Louis: C. V. Mosby, 1971.

Brunner, Lillian; Emerson, Charles; Ferguson, Kraeer; and Suddarth, Doris. *Textbook of Medical-Surgical Nursing.* 2nd ed. Philadelphia: J. B. Lippincott, 1970.

Ellenberg, Max, and Rifkin, Harold. *Diabetes Mellitus: Theory and Practice.* New York: McGraw Hill, 1970.

Gitman, Leo. "Diabetes Mellitus in the Aged," in U.S., Department of Health, Education, and Welfare, *Working with Older People—A Guide to Practice,* vol. 4, *Clinical Aspects of Aging,* Austin B. Chinn, ed. Washington, D.C.: U.S. Government Printing Office, 1971.

Mitchell, Helen; Rynbergen, Henderika; Anderson, Linnea; and Dibble, Marjorie. *Cooper's Nutrition in Health and Disease.* 15th ed. Philadelphia: J. B. Lippincott, 1968.

Nickerson, Donna. "Teaching the Hospitalized Diabetic." *American Journal of Nursing,* May 1972, p. 935.

Rosenthal, Helen, and Rosenthal, Joseph. *Diabetic Care in Pictures.* Philadelphia: J. B. Lippincott, 1968.

Rossman, Isadore. *Clinical Geriatrics.* Philadelphia: J. B. Lippincott, 1968.

Shuman, Charles R. *Recognition and Management of Diabetes in the Geriatric Patient.*

Smith, Dorothy; Germain, Carol; and Gips, Claudia. *Care of the Adult Patient.* 3rd ed. Philadelphia: J. B. Lippincott, 1971.

Weller, Charles, and Boylan, Brian. *The New Way to Live with Diabetes.* Garden City, N.Y.: Doubleday, 1966.

12

Restorative Nursing of Patients with Cancer

According to present statistics, cancer is the second leading cause of death in the United States. The American Cancer Society estimates that about 53 million people living at the present time will eventually contract this disease. Over half of those patients diagnosed as having cancer are over the age of sixty-five. Malignancies are also the second leading cause of hospitalization in elderly patients. Since older persons usually have other disabilities as well as the malignancy, rehabilitation and restoration of health is not a simple process. Not only the present illness, but also other existing diseases, which have an important influence, must be taken into account, if individualized restorative nursing care is to be given. A brief review of cancer—what it is and theories of its cause, diagnosis, and treatment—will be followed by specific principles of restorative nursing of elderly patients who have a malignancy in the body sites in which cancer is most prevalent.

CANCER REVIEW

Many lay persons associate the word "tumor" with the dread word "cancer," but tumors are not necessarily cancerous. Tumors, or abnormal growth of cells, are classified into two categories: benign and malignant. The cells in a benign tumor are uniform in size and shape and grow slowly. They do not invade surrounding tissue; rather they remain localized at a given area of the body. When the tumor is removed, it does not usually reappear. Also, these cells do not spread to other parts of the body. In malignant tumors, however, the cells differ in size and shape from the cells of the normal surrounding tissue from which they are derived. Malignant tumors usually grow rapidly, invading surrounding tissue, and these abnormal cells may travel from the original site to other locations in the body. The cells are transported by the lymphatic and/or circulatory systems and form secondary growths at body sites far from the primary area. This process is called metastasis. Unfortunately, the removal of the malignant tumor does not guarantee that it will not reappear. Cancer is a term used to describe a large number of diseases involving the spread of abnormal malignant cells.

Although the cause for this growth and spread of abnormal cells is unknown, there are many theories. Researchers throughout the world are constantly engaged in experiments which, hopefully, will unlock the secret to the cause or causes of these related diseases. There are many factors that appear to influence the incidence of some kinds of cancer. For example, prolonged exposure to the sun is probably a factor in the incidence of skin cancer. Those whose employment causes them to spend a great deal of time out of doors, such as fishermen, construction workers, and farmers, are more prone to skin cancer than office workers. Another theory is that constant irritation and trauma of tissues are factors in the development of cancer. Cancer of the lip is more likely to occur among individuals who smoke a pipe than among those who do not. The heat of the pipe and the irritation caused by rubbing the pipestem against the lip can be precipitating factors. Heredity may also play a role in the incidence of cancer. Some families seem to have hereditary tendencies for some form of cancer. For example, family histories reveal evidence of breast, uterine, or rectal malignancies. The relationship, however, of hereditary influence upon the incidence of cancer remains vague. Some precancerous conditions, especially polyps of the colon, tend to appear in several members of one family group.

Another theory which has had considerable publicity in recent years, is that of a virus as a cause of cancer. Although viruses have been introduced into the tissues of experimental animals and malignant tumors have resulted, the existence of a relationship between human cancer and a virus has not been proved.

Although the cause or causes of cancer remain unknown, we do know that there are sites within the body where malignancies tend to be more prevalent. Figure 12-1 indicates the percentage of incidence at each site according to sex.

The key to successful treatment is, of course, early detection. Since 50 percent of all cancer victims are senior citizens, it is particularly important for the elderly to practice the safeguards listed by the American Cancer Society. These safeguards include:

1. Reduce cigarette smoking or, if possible, abstain completely.
2. Have routine annual or semiannual physical examinations, including an oral inspection and proctoscopic examination, and for women, a pelvic examination and Papanicolaou test.
3. Perform a monthly self-examination of the breasts.
4. Avoid excessive exposure to the sun.

Routine physical examinations are a must for this age group—not a luxury that only the rich can afford. Local chapters of the American Cancer Society, cooperating with local medical groups, sponsor free clinics where various tests such as Pap smears are given. The nurse, as a member of the community, plays an important role in encouraging senior citizens to take advantage of such opportunities and in explaining and clarifying the seven warning signels of cancer. (See list.) These are an indication that a trip to the doctor is of immediate importance. The older adult will need encouragement, even prodding, along with emotional support. Afraid of what the doctor will find, the individual often puts off the visit until the symptoms become so severe that he is forced to seek help. Unfor-

---

CANCER'S 7 WARNING SIGNALS

C hange in bowel or bladder habits

A sore that does not heal

U nusual bleeding or discharge

T hickening or lump in breast or elsewhere

I ndigestion or difficulty in swallowing

O bvious change in wart or mole

N agging cough or hoarseness

If YOU have a warning signal, see your doctor!

tunately, if he waits too long, the malignancy may progress to the point where little, if any, treatment will prove effective. Therefore, the individual must get medical attention as early as possible. Support from his spouse and children may be necessary to provide the extra push needed to get him to seek help.

Ideally, the possibility of a malignancy will be picked up during a routine physical examination before symptoms have been noticed. A definite diagnosis of cancer is made through the examination of suspected tissue under a microscope. Removal of tissue from the suspicious area for this examination is called a biopsy. If the patient has not had routine physical examinations but has waited for symptoms to appear before making the visit to the doctor, his history and symptoms will provide clues as to the area involved. Sometimes the physician can see or feel the lesion.

Once a positive diagnosis is made, the method of treatment depends on whether or not there is a chance for cure. If the cancer has already metastasized to other vital structures, treatment will be based on relieving pain and the complications that arise rather than on trying to remove the cancerous tissues. This is called palliative treatment. The only true cure for cancer is the total removal or destruction of the abnormal cancer tissue, which may be accomplished through surgery, radiation, drug therapy, or a combination of these. For a complete review of these methods refer to a standard medical-surgical nursing text.

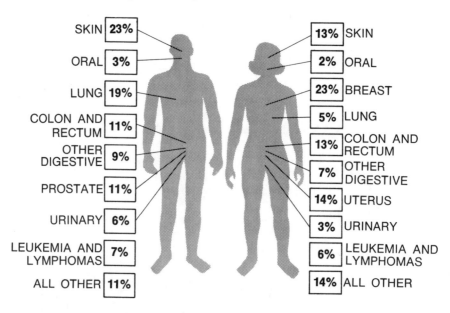

Figure 12-1:   Cancer incidence by site and sex. *(American Cancer Society)*

Approximately 50 percent of all cancers are now curable. Cancer is said to be cured if it is completely removed or destroyed and does not return to the original site or another location during the five-year period following destruction or removal. This is called a five-year survival.

The nurse, as a knowledgeable member of the community, can assist in special educational programs to increase the public's awareness of cancer and to dispel the notion that it can be cured through methods other than bona fide medical treatment.

RESTORATIVE NURSING

The patient who has undergone cancer surgery will have two major problems during the postoperative period. The first will be an alteration of his body image, and the second will be fear. The depth of these problems will be determined by the type, site, and extent of the surgery. Restorative nursing will focus on providing emotional support for the patient and his family and helping the patient to return to as nearly normal functioning as possible.

Much of the initial phase of restorative nursing is initiated in the acute general hospital and is continued in the patient's own home. Sometimes he is completely alone at home, without medical assistance, and left to flounder for himself. The need for the patient to be referred to the public health nursing agency and other agencies cannot be overstated. No one should have to cope with a first colostomy irrigation at home alone.

Two surgical procedures common among the older adult population are the colostomy and ileostomy. Both require that the patient receive specialized restorative nursing care.

COLOSTOMY

When part of the patient's colon is removed, he can no longer have bowel movements through the anus. An artificial opening on the abdomen is created—a colostomy—which permits elimination of feces from the remaining colon. This new opening is called a stoma. Since the stoma contains no muscle, the patient will not have control over it, and his most immediate concern will be, "How will I manage without that control?"

Initially, the person who has had a colostomy, or the colostomate, will have to wear a colostomy bag, which will collect the flow of material from the remaining portion of the colon. Unless the patient has a wet colostomy, he will be able to empty the colon after irrigating it. The irrigation is simply an enema through the stoma. This procedure should be scheduled at the patient's convenience—not the nurse's. Since it will take forty to sixty minutes for complete evacuation, the irrigation should be done when the bathroom is free. The specific procedure will be taught in the hospital, and the patient should be able to do it himself when he is discharged. Since the physical layout will be different in the patient's home, the public health nurse may have to assist the patient in making necessary adjustments. Some patients will be able to establish a pattern of evacuation that is so regular they will no longer need to wear a bag. A gauze bandage covering the stoma will be sufficient.

Activities are not limited. The usual sports and hobbies will be permitted, and travel is no problem for the colostomate. He will simply have to pack a small suitcase containing his irrigation equipment and other essential supplies.

The dietary intake can influence the regularity and consistency of the stools. Therefore, the patient is advised to follow a low residue diet during the postoperative period. Gradually, the diet will be more varied as new foods are added. The effects of these foods on the functioning of the bowel will need to be watched. Generally, patients have difficulty with hard-to-digest foods, such as corn on the cob, popcorn, celery, cole slaw, and coconut. Loose stools and gas can occur from eating beans, cabbage, broccoli, raw fruit, and highly spiced foods. Beer may cause flatus and diarrhea.

ILEOSTOMY

When the colon has been completely removed, all gastrointestinal elimination will be accomplished through an ileostomy stoma. Formerly, the colon handled all waste products, extracting water from the material, solidifying the waste, and storing it until elimination. The digestive enzymes produced in the ileum were also neutralized by the colon. Since these functions are no longer performed by the colon, the patient will have constant drainage from the ileostomy stoma. The fluid drainage will eventually become semisolid in nature, when the small intestine begins to absorb water into the body. The drainage must be kept off the skin, since it contains digestive enzymes that will cause skin breakdown. As with the colostomy, the patient will have no control over the elimination process. The ileostomate must wear a bag for the rest of his life. Many types of appliances are available to collect the drainage and to keep it off the skin. Karaya gum powder or karaya washers will prevent the discharge from attacking the skin.

Usually, the patient is not limited in his activities, and even swimming is permitted. Certainly, the patient will need to make some adjustments when performing these activities, but they can be done.

The diet is essentially the same as for the patient with colostomy. In addition, however, the patient will require large quantities of fluid and often increased amounts of salt.

Odor and gas are two concerns of the ileostomate. Certain foods may cause these problems. Experimentation with the diet will help the patient determine the culprit causing the odor. The physician can order oral medication to help reduce odor and flatus. A variety of deodorants for inside the pouch and room sprays are available, but the best odor barrier is the proper appliance.

Both the colostomate and the ileostomate have many questions, problems, and emotional upsets. Often the patient is so overwhelmed by the extent of his surgery that he cannot absorb all the information that is essential for living with his ostomy.

There are many people who are willing to help the ostomate and his family, including his physician, nurse, and other ostomates. More than 14,000 people belong to the United Ostomy Association. These individuals help each other and new ostomates with day-to-day problems. Members will visit patients in the hospital and at home to provide support and realistic advice about living with an ostomy. The address of the nearest ostomy group may be obtained by writing to the United Ostomy Association, 1111 Wilshire Blvd., Los Angeles, Calif., 90017. Other agencies, such as the local visiting nurse association and the homemaker service, will also provide concrete advice and assistance for the patient.

LARYNGECTOMY

The patient who awakens from general anesthesia following a laryngectomy, or the removal of his larynx, finds that his breathing, speaking, and swallowing abilities have been greatly altered. He is unable to speak, because of the removal of his vocal folds and voice box (larynx), and his breathing, coughing, and sneezing are performed through a tracheostomy, or an opening into his trachea. Immediately after the surgery intensive skilled nursing care will be required to keep the patient's tracheal stoma free of secretions, and to prevent occlusion and strangulation. During this period the patient will have a nasogastric tube in order to receive gavage feedings. After a few days the feeding tube is removed, and the patient progresses from soft foods to a full diet. (See Figure 12-2.)

Many patients are infuriated by the inability to speak, and they may express their feelings through nonverbal communications (throwing things, crying, refusing to see their spouse or family). A magic slate is usually given to the patient for written communication.

The patient depends on the nurse to remove all secretions from the tracheostomy, and he may be obsessed by the fear of choking to death during the immediate postoperative period.

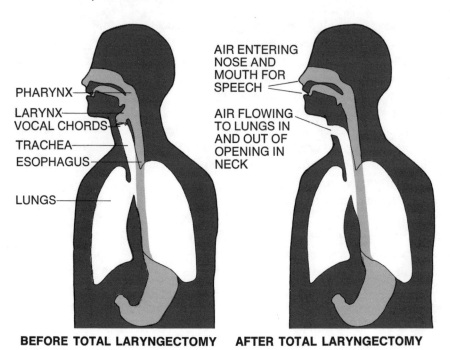

PHARYNX

LARYNX
VOCAL CHORDS

TRACHEA

ESOPHAGUS

LUNGS

AIR ENTERING
NOSE AND
MOUTH FOR
SPEECH

AIR FLOWING
TO LUNGS IN
AND OUT OF
OPENING IN
NECK

BEFORE TOTAL LARYNGECTOMY   AFTER TOTAL LARYNGECTOMY

Figure 12-2: Before and after a total laryngectomy.

When the patient is in the initial postoperative period, he should be visited by another laryngectomee—one who has successfully adjusted to his surgery and who has learned to speak again. This visitor will use esophageal speech, a technique that will be taught to the patient. In esophageal speech the patient takes air into the mouth and swallows or forces it into the esophagus. He then locks the air in place by holding his tongue to the roof of his mouth. When he forces the air back up, the walls of the esophagus and pharynx vibrate, and the air held in these passages vibrates also, causing low-pitched speech. The air is "belched" or "burped" back up, and the patient uses his mouth, teeth, and tongue to form words. Speech therapy is usually started when the muscles and mucous membrane surrounding the operative site are well healed. Therapy, of course, is ordered by the physician. The patient does not have to be hospitalized to participate in the therapy program. He may travel to a speech-and-hearing clinic, or a visiting speech therapist may give home instruction. Learning esophageal speech is a difficult task. Some patients learn quite readily; others may take as long as a year.

The advantage of esophageal speech is that it is ever present and does not make the stoma obvious. However, the patient may wish to use an artificial speech device, which is held against the neck and causes vibrations to occur, thereby permitting speech. Of course, the main disadvantage of an artificial larynx is that it calls attention to the patient's handicap.

The American Cancer Society has helped to sponsor the International Association of Laryngectomees which has, as its major purpose, the rehabilitation of laryngectomees. Further information about this association and the address of the local Laryngectomee Club or Lost Chord Club may be obtained from the International Society of Laryngectomees, 219 East 42nd Street, New York, New York 10017.

When the patient returns home, he will need to know how to care for the stoma himself. As early as possible the hospital nurse should teach the patient to care for his own laryngectomy set. He will be taught to remove the inner laryngectomy tube, cleanse it, and reinsert it. The outer cannula should never be removed except by the physician. The tubes should be handled with care. Usually, they are made of metal, and if they are dropped and dented, they will not fit together properly.

The stoma is covered with a small dressing or bib, which prevents mucus (expelled during coughing and sneezing) from staining the patient's clothing. This bib also helps to filter the air entering the lower respiratory tract, since the mucous membrane and the cilia of the nose, pharynx, and larynx no longer perform this function. The laryngectomee will feel most uncomfortable in dry, smoke-filled rooms. Moistening the bib will help relieve this discomfort. Sleeping will be easier if a vaporizer or humidifier is used all night. Air conditioning is difficult for the patient to tolerate, because the frigid air goes directly into the lungs without being warmed by the upper respiratory passages. The patient's taste and smell may be altered immediately after the operation, but he can be reassured that these senses will return quite satisfactorily.

All laryngectomees are concerned about their appearance, but it is not really a problem. The usual shirt and necktie will cover the stoma, although the shirt is altered to allow the patient to wipe away mucus that collects during coughing. The second button of the shirt is removed, and the button hole is sewed up. The shirt looks normal, but in reality has a convenient opening for cleaning the stoma. Both men and women can wear ascots or scarves with open-necked shirts. Turtle-neck or high-necked dresses will hide the stoma, and certain types of filigreed jewelry may be worn with a décolleté neckline.

After four to six weeks the stoma is sufficiently healed for the tracheostomy tubes to be removed. The tubing is left out for several hours each day, and after the patient has begun to breathe normally through the tubeless stoma, the tubing is permanently removed.

Patients should be able to resume most normal activities. Laryngectomees should not, however, lift heavy objects or resume activities that require hard straining, since they cannot hold in their breath as before.

The patient must carry some identification stating that he is a laryngectomee. If he should be in an accident, first aid such as mouth-to-mouth breathing or clearing an airway would have to be performed in a highly specialized manner. The standard identification card from the International Association of Laryngectomees includes specific instructions to rescuers and the name of the person to be notified in the event of an emergency. (See Figure 12-3.)

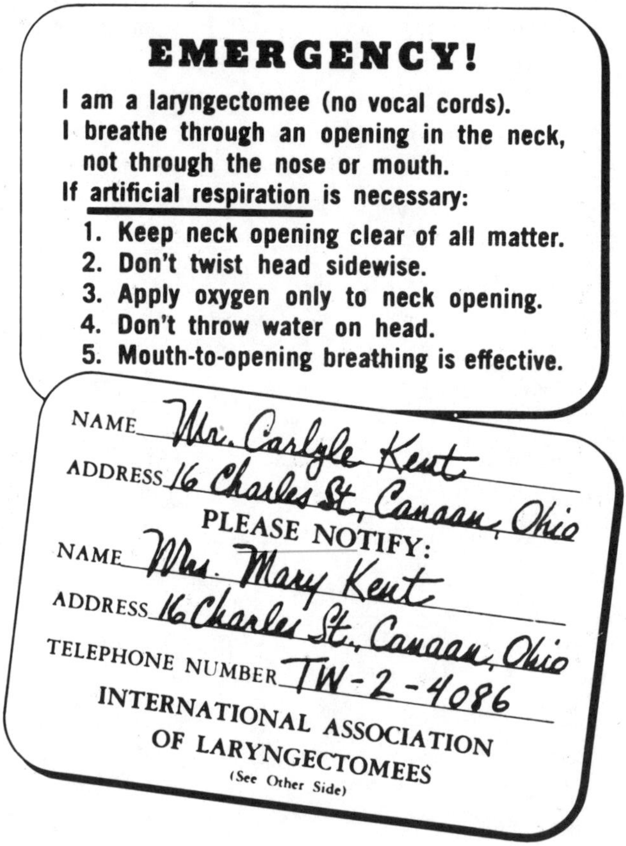

EMERGENCY!

I am a laryngectomee (no vocal cords).
I breathe through an opening in the neck, not through the nose or mouth.
If artificial respiration is necessary:

1. **Keep neck opening clear of all matter.**
2. **Don't twist head sidewise.**
3. **Apply oxygen only to neck opening.**
4. **Don't throw water on head.**
5. **Mouth-to-opening breathing is effective.**

NAME Mr. Carlyle Kent
ADDRESS 16 Charles St., Canaan, Ohio
PLEASE NOTIFY:
NAME Mrs. Mary Kent
ADDRESS 16 Charles St., Canaan, Ohio
TELEPHONE NUMBER TW-2-4086
INTERNATIONAL ASSOCIATION OF LARYNGECTOMEES
(See Other Side)

Figure 12-3: Official identification cards may be obtained from the International Association of Laryngectomees, 219 E. 42nd St., N. Y. 10017.

The patient should be careful not to get water in the stoma when taking a shower. In fact, a special shield can be used to cover the stoma so that water does not enter. The laryngectomee should tell barbers and beauticians to be very careful when shampooing, powdering, and in particular, using hair spray. These substances could be directly inhaled into the lung and cause severe respiratory difficulties. Swimming, of course, can never be permitted, for the patient could drown almost immediately.

Despair on the part of the laryngectomee—and his family is not unusual. What can the nurse do to help? First and foremost, she must listen to the family and pay attention to the patient when he tries to whisper to her, writes to her, or gestures at her. The nurse should also encourage the physician to contact the local Laryngectomy Club and arrange for a member to visit the patient. If no such club exists in the community, the local unit of the American Cancer Society will know of someone who will try to help the patient and his family. Even patients who have been unable to speak for years can be helped by these clubs.

Finally, the nurse can help the patient to learn to speak by encouraging him to use what he has learned in speech therapy. If there is no speech therapist in the community, the local Cancer Society may be able to suggest some qualified person nearby. Some school systems employ speech therapists who aid children with speech difficulties. Perhaps this person could be of aid to the patient.

RADICAL MASTECTOMY

Immediately following a mastectomy, or the removal of the patient's breast, the patient will need to be observed closely for shock and hemorrhage. A large area of the chest will be bandaged, and this will be frightening to the patient. The dressings may be quite snug, and the patient's arm may be bandaged across the chest in order to give added pressure to the dressing, which may be upsetting. She should be told why pressure dressings are used and that some drainage from the operative site is expected. Good postoperative nursing care based on principles of restorative nursing for immobilized patients is now indicated.

The first few days the patient's arm (on the operative side) may be placed in a sling when she is out of bed. This *does not* mean, however, that this arm should always be at rest. In fact, quite the opposite is true. As soon as possible after surgery, sometimes within twenty-four hours, active exercise is initiated. Each day the patient should do more and more of her own activities of daily living (using the arm on the affected side). Hair brushing is an especially good exercise. Examples of other appropriate exercises are shown in Figure 12-4.

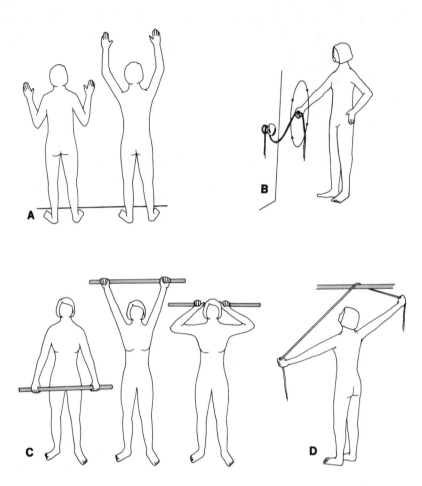

Figure 12-4: The purpose of the exercise program is to secure a complete range of motion of the affected shoulder joint. (Adapted from Radler: A Handbook for Your Recovery. New York, The Society of Memorial Center)   **A.** *Wall handclimbing.* Stand facing wall, with feet apart. Bend elbows and place palms on the wall at shoulder level. By flexing the fingers, work hands up the wall until arms are fully extended. Reverse procedure.   **B.** *Rope turning.* Stand facing door. Take free end of light rope in hand of the operated side. Place other hand on hip. With arm extended and held away from body—nearly parallel with floor—turn rope, making as wide swings as possible. Slow at first—speed up later.   **C.** *Rod or Broom.* Grasp rod with both hands, held about 2 feet apart. With arms straight, raise rod over head. Bend elbows, lowering rod behind head. Reverse maneuver.   **D.** *Pulley.* Toss rope over shower curtain rod or doorway curtain rod. Stand as nearly under rope as possible. Grasp an end in each hand. Extend arms straight and away from body. Pull left arm up by tugging down with right arm, and vice versa.

The purpose of muscle retraining is to prevent a contracture, promote use of the limb, and reduce the lymphedema. The patient must use proper posture while performing these exercises, and she will need to be aware of her posture because the shoulder on the affected side will tend to droop. Exercise and conscious efforts to improve her posture will help. All exercises should be performed with both arms, as illustrated in Figure 12-4.

When the patient is discharged, she may be completely overwhelmed by the very thought of changing her own dressings. Of course, she should have learned how to change the dressing before the discharge. Still, just to look at the incision may be more than she can bear, and the visiting nurse can be an invaluable friend and assistant to the patient, helping her over a difficult emotional hump. Moreover, the visiting nurse can report the healing process to the surgeon.

The patient may be anxious about her physical appearance. Eventually she can be fitted for a prosthesis, but until that time other measures will have to be utilized. Many women who have had this surgery find that a stretch sleep bra or nighttime bra is most comfortable during this interim period. Soft material such as lamb's wool or cotton may be used to pad this brassiere. The nurse can contact the local Cancer Society to arrange for a volunteer who has successfully recovered from a mastectomy to visit the patient. The volunteer can aid the patient in restoring her normal physical appearance, in adjusting to increasing activities, and in selecting a permanent prosthesis. Although there are expert fitters in the business of prosthetic breasts, the most helpful person is one who has been through the experience herself.

A mastectomy need not be totally devastating to the patient—emotionally or physically. Restorative nursing plays a major role in helping patients to make a positive postoperative adjustment to this surgery.

WHAT ABOUT TELLING THE PATIENT THE DIAGNOSIS?

It is always the prerogative of the physician to decide when, what, and how much to tell the patient and his family. In many cases the surgeon will tell the patient that he suspects the presence of malignancy. This is done in an attempt to prepare the patient emotionally for the possibility of a colostomy, ileostomy, laryngectomy, radical mastectomy, or other extensive surgical procedure. Some patients may even sign preoperative permits that specify the exact nature of the surgery. Special permits are also needed for X ray, radium, and other types of radiation therapy. Usually, the patient senses that there is something seriously wrong with him, and he will question his family, the nurse, chaplain, doctors, and so on. The doctor, and only the doctor (never the nurse), tells the patient about his illness—its nature, extent, and prognosis. The nurse must know what the physician has told the patient, so that she can continue to give him emotional support on the basis of this information.

PROGNOSIS

The prognosis depends on the site, type, extent, and infiltration of the malignancy. The prognosis may be excellent or the patient's remaining lifetime may be limited to a few months. Cancer, however, is not synonymous with death. More patients are cured today than in the past, due to earlier diagnosis and treatment of this disease.

RESEARCH

Vast research projects are being conducted to determine the cause of, and a cure for, cancer. Meanwhile, until this research bears significant results, studies are being carried out on the use and effects of various drugs and other methods of treatment. Certain drugs have been particularly effective in halting or slowing down the growth of certain types of malignant cells. The discovery and use of antineoplastic drugs and radioactive substances are the result of recent research projects. Such scientific inquiry is funded by the United States federal government, the American Cancer Society, the Leukemia Society, and other private and public agencies. Some nations have joined together in their search for a cancer cure. These international efforts are recent developments in joint cooperative ventures, and it is indeed encouraging to know that a worldwide research battle is being waged against cancer.

All people look to the medical researchers for a solution to the problem of cancer. There is always the hope that a cure is just around the corner. It is this hope that gives us a reason for trying, for fighting, for tolerating all of the problems associated with the disease. Thus, research, with its ever present look to the future, supports us all.

STUDY QUESTIONS AND PROBLEMS

1. The local unit of the American Cancer Society is sponsoring a screening day for senior citizens. The testing will include sigmoidoscopy for all and a Pap smear for the women. The testing will be performed at local hospitals, and the Red Cross will provide transportation to and from the testing center. Your neighbors do not understand these tests and their implications. How would you explain the procedures and why they are so important?
2. Visit the local unit of the American Cancer Society and review its materials for professional personnel and patients. What services does the unit provide for cancer patients?

3. Mrs. Mendes has returned to her home following a radical mastectomy. Since there is no visiting nurse in the community, she has asked you, her friend, to help her at home. Develop a plan of care for her that includes exercise of the affected side and the resumption of household duties.

BIBLIOGRAPHY

Adler, Sal. "Speech After Laryngectomy." *American Journal of Nursing,* October 1969, p. 2138.

After Mastectomy. New York: American Cancer Society, 1970.

Aliapoulios, M. A., and Gribbons, Carol A. "Treatment for Advanced Breast Carcinoma." *American Journal of Nursing,* May 1972, p. 678.

Barckley, Virginia. "A Visiting Nurse Specializes in Cancer Nursing." *American Journal of Nursing,* August 1970, p. 1681.

Brunner, Lillian; Emerson, Charles; Ferguson, Kraeer; and Suddarth, Doris. *Textbook of Medical-Surgical Nursing.* 2nd ed. Philadelphia: J. B. Lippincott, 1970.

Cancer Facts and Figures. New York: American Cancer Society, 1973.

Cancer of the Breast. New York: American Cancer Society, 1969.

Craytor, Josephine. "Talking with Persons Who Have Cancer." *American Journal of Nursing,* May 1969, p. 744.

Gibbs, Gertrude, and White, Marilyn. "Stomal Care." *American Journal of Nursing,* February 1972, p. 268.

Gribbons, Carol, and Aliapoulios, M. A. "Early Carcinoma of the Breast." *American Journal of Nursing,* September 1969, p. 1945.

Gutkowski, Frances. "Ostomy Procedure: Nursing Care Before and After." *American Journal of Nursing,* February 1972, p. 262.

Harrell, Helen C. "To Lose a Breast." *American Journal of Nursing,* May 1972, p. 676.

International Association of Laryngectomees. Sponsored by the American Cancer Society, *Helping Words for the Laryngectomee.* New York: International Association of Laryngectomees, 1964.

International Association of Laryngectomees. Sponsored by the American Cancer Society, *Rehabilitating Laryngectomees.* New York: International Association of Laryngectomees, 1970.

Katona, Elizabeth A. "Learning Colostomy Control." *American Journal of Nursing,* March 1967, p. 534.

———. *Managing Your Colostomy So a Normal Life Is Yours Again.* (A professional aid for the new colostomate). Chicago: Hollister, 1971.

———. *Managing Your Ileostomy So It Doesn't Manage You.* (A professional aid for the new Ileostomate). Chicago: Hollister, 1971.

New York City Cancer Committee. *Essentials of Cancer Nursing.* New York: American Cancer Society, 1963.

13

Death and Dying

Our culture has built up practices that tend to soften or disguise the reality of death. Funeral homes have "slumber rooms," and the art of embalming is so sophisticated that those viewing the body remark that the deceased looks better than he ever did. Some persons are now requesting that, upon death, their bodies undergo a deep-freezing technique that will preserve them so that they can be thawed years from now, when a cure for the cause of death has been found. All these situations are examples of a denial of death. Our youth-oriented culture, particularly, has difficulty in dealing with the idea that life as we know it must come to an end. Western man has long looked in vain for the fountain of youth. In those fleeting moments when each of us thinks of death, we seem to think of another's death, not our own. Deep down inside we know death will occur, but on the surface we dismiss the thought.

The attitudes people have toward death come from a variety of sources—religious philosophy, culture, family concepts, and one's personal experience with death. According to the Judeo-Christian concept, death is a bridge between life on earth and unity with God in an afterlife. Although the body dies, the soul of man lives on. Death is a fulfillment of life rather than an abrupt end. In some Oriental cultures people believe the human soul joins the world of its ancestors, and worship and homage to one's ancestors is an important part of the culture. The ancient Egyptians and later the Vikings provided their dead with food, clothing, and other items necessary for the deceased to make the journey to the next land.

Primitive cultures assert that man will travel to his forefathers, becoming one with his ancestors as a link in the chain between life and death. Thus, one's cultural and religious philosophy provide a framework within which his personal experiences with death take on meaning.

Ethnic, community, and family patterns in dealing with death are as different as one family is from another. Just as life is highly individualized, so are attitudes toward death and dying. These attitudes are also colored by the experiences the individual has had with friends and relatives who have died. Whether these experiences were positive or negative will, in large part, influence one's ability to deal with his own death and the death of others.

UNDERSTANDING DEATH AND DYING

One's ability to face the reality of death and dying depends on his own personality, his life-style, and his ability to cope with other crises in his life. Unless the nurse devotes time to resolving her conflicts regarding death, and unless she gives some thought to her own views on the subject, it will be difficult for her to meet the needs of a dying patient. Of course, it is not easy to resolve personal conflicts about death, and the task cannot be accomplished in a short period.

Many books and magazine articles have been written on the subject of death and dying. Many authors agree that the dying patient goes through a series of emotional stages before the final phase of acceptance. Research has shown that the dying person's emotional reaction can be divided into five major phases. The first phase is one of rejection—a denial of the possibility of death. ("It can't be me.") As this first reaction wanes, the second reaction is usually one of anger, as if the patient were saying, "Why is it my turn?" This anger is vented against loved ones and those in close contact with the person. If the patient is hospitalized, the nursing staff will take the brunt of this anger and hostility. The next stage comes when, having lost his anger, the patient begins to bargain with his God for more time. This is a personal, private affair. "Just give me another year to finish my unfinished business." When this third phase is completed, a period of depression results in which the inescapable reality is clearly seen. The patient quietly withdraws into himself. This is a preparation for the final stage of acceptance and the development of an attitude of "My life has been fulfilled —I am ready." Not all patients go through these five stages, however. Some overlapping may occur. The patient may revert to a previous stage, instead of following an orderly progression, or his life may be terminated before the final stage of acceptance.

Many articles give examples of children and young people who are terminally ill and tell of the emotional turmoil caused by their illnesses. Their stories are heartrending. With the aged, however, the story is not quite so dramatic. Their emotional and physical care presents essentially the same problems, but will be modified to meet the special needs of the older adult. Generally, elderly patients state that they don't mind dying, but are afraid of the act of dying. This act may be feared because it is unknown or because the patient is afraid of a painful, agonizing death. The independent person may fear total dependency, helplessness, and loss of control over himself. A very real fear is that of dying alone. Usually, the important events of one's life include others—relatives and friends sharing one's joys, sorrows, and anxieties. No wonder the dying person seeks someone, perhaps anyone, who will share his final act. It need not be the intellectual, articulate person who has all the proper words, but certainly it must be someone who cares.

The importance of preparing patients psychologically for all sorts of events (physical examinations, treatments, surgery, etc.) is emphasized in all educational programs for nursing personnel. Yet the nurse is often ill-equipped to help her patients prepare for the ultimate act of living—dying. Psychiatric nursing concepts include listening to the patient, accepting the patient as he is, and creating an atmosphere of openness so that communication can take place. But when the patient says, "I know I haven't much longer to live," the nurse's standard response may be, "Oh, don't talk that way. You'll be fine!" This response, in addition to stifling further communication, shows that the nurse is having difficulty accepting the reality of death. Perhaps the problem is compounded by the belief that this emotional aspect should be left to the specialist—the priest, minister, or rabbi. Although religious consolation is the province of the clergy, the nurse's day-to-day contact with the patient provides a real opportunity for her to give the emotional support necessary between visits from the clergy.

In order to plan for the patient's physical and emotional supportive care, the nurse must learn as much about him as possible. Since the patient will deal with this experience as he has dealt with others in the past, the nurse's goal is to help the dying patient to be as comfortable as possible, as he faces dying in his own way. He will need support—physical, emotional, and religious—from the nurse, doctor, chaplain, and his family. The family may also provide information about the patient's cultural attitudes, lifestyle, and religious and philosophical convictions. Nursing personnel should be alert to indications of the patient's readiness to talk about death. To many patients death means a final peace—no more concerns, no more pain. Others may be resigned—"I can't fight anymore. I'm too tired."

The vast majority of elderly patients die in an institution. The home environment with familiar faces and cherished possessions has been replaced by an impersonal setting. How frightening to be dependent on strangers when facing death. How lonely it must be to have the nurse reject you when all you want to do is talk and have someone listen. If, in an effort to handle her own feelings, the nurse withdraws from this emotionally painful situation, she leaves the patient alone and further isolated.

The nurse must decide just what role she can play in the care of this dying patient. The determination of her role will come from her attitudes toward death, and she must understand her feelings about death. Does death cause her to feel she has failed as a restorer of health and well-being? Does death remind her of her own mortality? Does death renew her feelings of inadequacy and inability to care for the dying patient? If she views death as a defeat, then she gives in to frustration and helplessness. She may unintentionally withdraw from everything except the essentials of the patient's physical care, or she may submerge herself in "doing for the patient," as if to reduce the opportunity to just sit, talk, and listen. Her physical presence may be at the bedside, but her emotional presence will be elsewhere. She may use complicated terminology to avoid discussing any threatening subject with her patient. She may not talk to the patient or his family at all.

The nurse must then decide whether or not she is going to help herself and this patient and his family. It would be unreasonable for each and every nurse to think she can effectively care for the dying patient. If a nurse has recently had a death in her immediate family, she may not be able to care for dying patients until a later time. Or her recent bereavement may have increased her awareness and ability to understand the patient and his family. All nurses should come to terms with themselves regarding their feelings about death and dying patients. Death occurs in all clinical areas, swiftly or slowly, and the nurse cannot avoid this kind of care forever. Hopefully, if the nurse understands her own strengths and weaknesses in dealing with the dying patient and if she learns as much as she can about her patient, the patient's last days and hours can be ones in which his dignity is preserved.

CARE OF THE DYING

The focus throughout this text has been on the principles of returning function to the patient (that is, restorative nursing). Death, however, is opposed to all this restoring. When function cannot be returned to, or supported in the vital body structures, the process of dying has begun. The nurse should be able to recognize the signs of forthcoming death.

Progressive failure of vital body functions will indicate that death is approaching. The patient will be pale and covered with sweat, and he will breathe with difficulty through both his mouth and his nose. He will lose sensation and movement in the lower limbs. These problems will ascend gradually. This patient may require more skilled nursing care than one in active rehabilitation, since the person who is dying usually cannot express his needs or wants. Because he is mouth breathing, the oral mucosa and tongue will be exceedingly dry. Mouth care, including moistening of the oral tissues, is essential. The patient's attempts to swallow may cause him to choke, and he will have difficulty sipping through a straw. An ice chip or two may be placed between the patient's cheek and teeth to help keep the mouth moistened, or the nurse may place a few ice chips in a cloth or piece of gauze and let the patient suck on the ice. Once the nurse has found a method to maintain oral comfort, she may teach it to a family member. Very often distraught relatives sit by and feel useless and helpless. Usually they are most happy to assist in the care of a loved one. Weeping relatives and those who are sitting in the room fighting back their tears are usually grateful for an opportunity to do something that is helpful.

Most moribund patients appear to be in a comatose state. It is not certain whether or not the patient receives and interprets external stimuli through his sense organs. Many believe that a patient's inability to respond to verbal stimulation does not mean that he is unable to hear. For this reason communication between the patient and nurse, as well as the patient and his family, should be maintained. Communication will help to ensure personalized nursing care and to prevent the patient from becoming a "thing." As always, the nurse should inform the patient of her intentions before starting a nursing procedure. It is wise to assume that the patient will be able to hear and see what is very close to him. Therefore, the nurse should stand near the bed and speak distinctly, at a normal volume and speed. She should announce her arrivals and departures to the patient, and leave some lights on so that he can distinguish what is going on. Family members, too, should announce their comings and goings and inform the patient of their presence. A touch on the hand or shoulder, a smile, and a kiss from a loved one are all meaningful nonverbal communications that may well be understood by the patient.

Greater comfort will be afforded the dying patient if his position is changed frequently. Turning the patient on his side will help to ease labored respirations, and when he is on his side, drainage from his nose and mouth will be enhanced by simple gravity. Many patients find it easier to breathe when their shoulders and head are elevated.

Profuse sweating occurs, and the patient's skin becomes icy cold, due to a decrease in peripheral circulation. Some authors have reported that the patient does not complain about being cold. Rather, he complains about being unusually warm. Because he feels warm, the patient may begin to toss and turn in an effort to remove the bed linens and make himself cooler. Very weak patients may only have the strength to pull or pick at the sheets. The environment must be comfortable for the patient—a little cooler than usual. Sponging with tepid water will help to relieve the sweating and provide some cooling.

The sphincter muscles of the anus and urinary tract will become relaxed, and the patient may become incontinent without realizing it. A properly positioned urinal or bedpan will be genuinely appreciated by the patient. Skin care is essential, especially in the perineal area.

The patient may express a wish to see the chaplain. In most institutions there are clergy to meet the spiritual needs of Catholic, Protestant, and Jewish patients. If the patient does not have a priest, minister, or rabbi of his own, the nurse may suggest one of the institution's chaplains. The nurse should arrange her care plan to allow plenty of time for the chaplain's visit. Also, she should greet and welcome him as well as offer any assistance. Usually, the greatest need is uninterrupted quiet and privacy.

Spiritual needs should be met while the patient is conscious and alert. If the matter of religious consolation is not discussed by the patient or his family, the nurse may suggest that a clergyman visit the patient. Sometimes the family thinks that such a visit would be too upsetting to the patient. However, most dying patients are happy to see their clergyman, and they sincerely appreciate religious consolation. Sometimes the patient will not want the chaplain to visit, but will want the nurse or family to read the Bible or say some prayers. The nurse should try to find some time to sit with the patient and read to him as he wishes.

If a Catholic priest is to hear the patient's confession, everyone should leave the room, close the door, and wait to be called back. When the Sacrament of the Sick is to be given, the priest will appreciate some assistance. When this sacrament is administered, the priest anoints the patient's senses and prays for recovery. This is by no means the last rites; rather it is a sacrament of hope and life. When the patient is to receive the Holy Eucharist (Communion), the nurse should cover the bedside table with a white cloth and have a glass of water, a spoon, and a cloth napkin on the table. A lighted blessed candle (when oxygen is not in use) and a crucifix are also at the bedside. Most hospitals, nursing homes, and extended care facilities have a communion set, which contains all of the articles used to prepare for the priest's arrival with the Holy Eucharist.

Many times the family will ask the nurse about the patient's last stages, the so-called death agony. All who have worked with the dying will attest that there is no such thing as the death agony. Individuals who have been close to death and recovered say that they have no recollection of pain or unpleasant thoughts. Thus, the final stages are painless, with the patient in an unconscious sleeplike state from which he cannot be aroused.

Once the vital signs have ceased, the physician will pronounce the patient dead. If the patient has been sick a long time, the relatives may be greatly relieved now that it is all over. However, there may be an emotional outburst, and the nurse must understand and accept this behavior. In fact, she should understand that she may shed a few tears also.

Relatives should be allowed to see the patient one more time before they leave the hospital. Any apparatus around the patient, such as intravenous tubing and poles, catheters, or oxygen tents, should be removed first. This will help to reinforce the reality that the death has occurred and perhaps bring about the realization that the patient is at peace.

Don't just hand the family a little collection of the patient's belongings and dismiss them. It is not easy to lose a loved one, no matter how old he may have been, and the family needs support from the nurse. Offer them a place where they can sit and talk, offer them a glass of water or a cup of coffee, smile, and listen. The family will be bombarded with many questions and problems—Do they want an autopsy? Who will be the undertaker? How should they tell other family members? What kind of arrangements should they make? Don't let the family slip away from you. Walk them to the door, say good-bye, and add any personal comments that may be appropriate. Perhaps you, too, loved the patient and will miss him very much. Do tell the family. Such words of sympathy are very soothing.

Death is a reality that all must accept. The nurse cannot halt its progress within the patient, but she can protect him from impersonal care and from being reduced to an object. Through her specialized care she assists the patient in completing his final act—dying with dignity.

STUDY QUESTION

It has been six months since Mr. Porter's death, and his wife is now able to discuss her feelings about the hospital personnel. She says, "The nurse said, 'Go home. There is nothing you can do. I've seen so many people unconscious like that. He may last minutes or hours. Just go home.' "

Mrs. Porter continues, "I just wanted to be with him. He was all alone. What if he woke up and no one was there? I'll never know if he woke up and I wasn't there when he needed me."

Discuss Mrs. Porter's feelings. How could the nursing staff have helped while her husband was dying?

BIBLIOGRAPHY

Anonymous. "Notes of a Dying Professor." *The Pennsylvania Gazette,* March 1972, p. 18.

Burnside, Irene M. "The Patient I Didn't Want." *American Journal of Nursing,* August 1968, p. 1666.

Choron, Jacques. *Modern Man and Mortality.* New York: Macmillan, 1964.

Gordon, David Cole. *Overcoming the Fear of Death.* New York: Macmillan, 1970.

Gress, Lucille. "Sensitizing Students to the Aged." *American Journal of Nursing,* October 1971, p. 1968.

Hoffman, Esther. "Don't Give Up on Me." *American Journal of Nursing,* January 1971, p. 60.

Jaeger, Dorothea, and Simmons, Leo. *The Aged Ill.* New York: Appleton-Century-Crofts, 1970.

Jourard, Sidney. "Suicide: The Invitation to Die." *American Journal of Nursing,* February 1970, p. 269.

Kneisl, Carol. "Thoughtful Care for the Dying." *American Journal of Nursing,* March 1968, p. 550.

Kubler-Ross, Elisabeth. *On Death and Dying.* New York: Macmillan, 1971.

———. "What Is It Like to Be Dying?" *American Journal of Nursing,* January 1971, p. 54.

McNulty, Barbara J. "St. Christopher's Outpatients." *American Journal of Nursing,* December 1971, pp. 2328–2330.

Mervyn, Frances. "Plight of Dying Patients in Hospitals." *American Journal of Nursing,* October 1971, p. 1988.

Schoenberg, Bernard; Carr, Arthur; Peretz, David; Kutscher, Austin (editors). *Loss and Grief: Psychological Management in Medical Practice.* New York: Columbia University Press, 1970.

Sharp, Donna. "Lessons From a Dying Patient." *American Journal of Nursing,* July 1968, p. 1517.

Stevens, Peter. *Emotional Crisis.* New York: Odyssey Press, 1965.

Vaillot, Sister Madeleine Clemence. "Hope—The Restoration of Being." *American Journal of Nursing,* February 1970, p. 268.

Vervoerdt, Adriaan, and Wilson, Ruby. "Communication with Fatally Ill Patients—Tacit or Explicit?" *American Journal of Nursing,* November 1967, p. 2307.

Vischer, A. L. *On Growing Old.* Boston: Houghton Mifflin, 1967.

Worcester, Albert. *The Care of the Aged, the Dying, and the Dead.* Springfield, Illinois: Charles C. Thomas, 1961.

14

Looking Ahead

There is much speculation regarding what our world will be like in the twenty-first century. For one thing, excursions to the moon may become a reality; trips to other planets are not inconceivable. Cures for the leading causes of death may be found, causing the number of people reaching retirement age to increase still further. Hopefully, ways will be found to reverse the pollution of the air, water, and earth, so that our natural resources can be utilized and enjoyed without being exploited and abused.

What will the American life-style be like in future years, as an increasing number of technological advances take place? From time to time jokes are made about reversing the individual's working life and his retirement life. Wouldn't such a reversal have a profound effect on life-styles? Our youthful years would not be burdened with having to earn a living. We would have time to enjoy all those activities that now have to be crammed into weekends and an annual vacation. When this phase of life is completed, the later years could be devoted to active employment. Although this concept has certain desirable aspects, our society and its value systems would have to be completely revamped before it could even be considered, let alone implemented.

RETIREMENT IN THE FUTURE

The above thoughts are, of course, mere speculation, but one fact is upon us—the retirement age of sixty-two will be reduced by ten years in the foreseeable future. Unions and other organized employee groups are pro-

214

viding the impetus for this change. Soon there will be a normal employment span of thirty years and conceivably twenty-five to thirty years of retirement. Leisure time during the working years has already been increased for those who have a four-day workweek. The thought of a further reduction to a three-day workweek makes some wonder what they will ever do with all that time. With the shortened workweek plus the earlier retirement age, large numbers of *younger* Americans (semiretired or retired) will have an abundance of time on their hands.

By the year 2000, the characteristics of the older population will have changed. The average older adult will be more like the average middle-aged person of today. Most of them will be high school graduates and nearly half will have had some college education. More highly skilled than today's older adult, the retiree of the future will not be satisfied to idle away twenty-five to thirty years. Many will need assistance in planning for a meaningful life during these years.

Since we know that early retirement is fast approaching, one should make plans during his working years in anticipation of this fact. Planning includes many facets. The most obvious is that of economics. "How much money should I be saving and when should I begin?" Various kinds of retirement plans were discussed in Chapter 2. During the initial job interview, the nurse should ask her potential employer about the pension plan available to her. The young employee should not underestimate the important value of this fringe benefit. Other retirement plan information can be obtained from the organized employee group, a reliable insurance agent, the local bank, and the Social Security Administration Office.

Some people say that the key to a successful and happy retirement is the acquisition of many hobbies during the working years. The person who has devoted a lifetime to his job has nothing to fall back on when the job is no longer there. However, interests that are job-related can carry over into one's retirement years. Nurses, for example, are usually people-oriented and service-oriented, and retired nurses may find their contributions most welcome in community service organizations and other social service agencies. Activities in such service organizations serve a twofold purpose. They provide meaningful work and recreation. If one expands his interests during the employment years, the retirement years can be filled with fun and activity.

Society must also play a more dominant role in helping its citizens to prepare for retirement and in making these years more livable. The school's role in educating each citizen regarding later adulthood and retirement has not been a prominent one. Until very recently evening adult schools sponsored by local boards of education have been predominantly hobby-oriented. Some adult schools are changing to include job training and retraining. More needs to be done to educate our citizens for a life off the job as well as on the job. Local schools should offer preretirement education programs to help those who are approaching retirement to prepare for the future. As has been stated previously, industry and many unions now offer preretirement preparation and counseling for both worker and spouse. In the future, schools should participate more fully with local unions and management in the process of educating citizens in this phase of lifetime learning. In addition to helping pre-retirees to think and work through the basic considerations in retirement (finances, home location, etc.), these programs should assist them to determine what they want from life and how to achieve it. Keeping the mind active and functioning as well as maintaining social skills represents a new and important dimension in this educational process. Pre-retirement education represents one positive approach to retirement.

Schools should also play a leadership role by conducting lectures, discussion groups, and workshops for senior citizens, conducting seminars in consumer education, and helping widows by including lectures and discussions on such topics as adjusting to widowhood, insurance coverage, budgeting, bank accounts, and one's rights as a homeowner. Perhaps, as the stereotyped role of women in our society changes, widows will want and need courses with a different type of content. Courses for widowers may incorporate homemaking skills, which in the past have been stereotyped as being for women only.

As schools become more "community-focused," the senior citizen with special skills may well teach an essential aspect of education—how we grow and develop. This would be an integral part of the entire school curriculum and include biological, social, and emotional growth and development at the various stages of life—childhood, adolescence, adulthood, and late adulthood. The expertise of the senior citizen will be invaluable in bringing to the students real-life experiences and understanding. If the school is truly community-focused, students may have planned experiences with older people in nursing homes or senior citizen centers, which will provide an opportunity that cannot be gained within the four walls of a classroom. Both the young and the old benefit from this give and take, and hopefully mutual respect and understanding result.

CARE OF THE AGED IN THE FUTURE

One of the most consistent recommendations from the delegates in the special sessions of the 1971 White House Conference on Aging was that the elderly person remain in his own home for as long as possible. In order for this goal to be achieved, alternatives to institutional care must be developed and implemented.

Cities could be designed to meet the needs of the elderly. Such cities would have areas without curbing, and ramps instead of steps to assure easy access to all buildings. Such cities could be possible, if senior citizens could be a part of city planning. Today, many cities are working to rejuvenate their downtown shopping districts. An effective means of doing this has been to close the major streets to automobile traffic, thereby creating a pedestrian walkway and shopping area. With a little planning the rejuvenated downtown area could also be a safe and pleasant place for the elderly to shop and socialize. Economical and reliable public transportation would further enhance the project.

At the White House Conference on Aging in 1971, it was recommended that there should be a *multipurpose senior center* in every community or, when appropriate, in every neighborhood. These centers would provide basic social services and link all older persons to appropriate sources of help, including home-delivered services. The centers would be architecturally designed to meet the needs of the elderly, including safety, comfort, and easy access. Both indoor and outdoor areas would be included. The programs would include recreational activities such as arts and crafts, and meals would be available, at reasonable cost, in a pleasant dining room where appetites and conversation would be stimulated. An additional benefit would be nutritionally balanced meals.

It was recommended that three specific types of services be given by these centers: supportive services, preventive services, and protective services. The first, supportive services, would be those that help the older person to remain in his own home. Specifically, the center could arrange for homemaker–home health aide service, skilled nursing care, meals on wheels, and escort service. Preventive services, such as screening clinics, staffed by mental health workers, social workers, public health nurses, and special counselors, could detect problems before they develop and intervene when necessary. Protective services would include legal services and would enable the older person to guard his civil rights and personal welfare. The focus would be on meeting the needs of those in the most acute difficulty.

The center would also contain a government outreach office, where the older American could obtain information about Medicare, Social Security, and Food Stamps. The applications for these programs could be completed and returned to this office, which would save the older person from making trips all over the city to apply for these government programs. Other services would include a pharmacy, barber shop, beauty parlor, and chiropodist

—all at special reduced prices. Small stores, such as clothing stores, card shops, food stores, sandwich shops, designed to meet the shopping needs of the aged, could be a part of the center, too.

All of this would be of no avail to the aged person who is homebound due to a disability, however. He needs special services if he is to stay where he is. One of the best known services for those confined to the home is that of the homemaker–home health aide. People from this service carry out assigned tasks in the family's residence under the supervision of a professional, who assesses the need for service and implements the plan of care. It is estimated that there are only 30,000 homemaker–home health aides in the entire United States. They serve all categories of people in need: the ill, aged, disabled, children, and others with health and/or social problems. The number of homemaker–home health aides recommended to meet the present need is 300,000, or one aide per every 1,000 persons in the total population. For the senior citizen this ratio should be 1 aide per 100 people. Obviously, there is a need for the homemaker–home health aide service to be expanded. Not only are more aides needed, but the hours of service need to be more flexible, so that the aging person and his family can obtain full-time or part-time service, day or evening service. Related inhome services, such as meals on wheels, friendly visitors, shopping service, laundry service, chore services, and transportation service, need to be developed or expanded. In the rural community such services could be provided by mobile facilities, which would travel to the aged.

In both urban and rural areas public health nursing services will need to be expanded as more and more elderly persons are cared for at home. Opportunities for practical nurses in the visiting nurse service will become more abundant. Public health nurses, usually with the title of public health nursing coordinator, will visit institutionalized patients prior to their discharge to plan for their care at home.

As new and more effective methods of delivering health care emerge, the need for new kinds of health care workers will become apparent. Appropriate educational programs will need to be developed. Local hospitals will expand their services to the homebound elderly. Physicians (from the hospital) will be assigned to home care and will work with the other personnel currently giving patient care.

Live-in companions and the aged person may be matched—much like computer dating today. A night sitter program would allow the elderly person's family to have an evening of entertainment and diversion.

When institutionalization is necessary, the older person will still be served by the community. It is anticipated that special programs, enabling the resident to participate in community activities, will take place in the institution. Thus, the resident will not become an isolated nonentity.

The services of the nursing home may be spread to the community through some direct services at home, walk-in services (such as meals), or teaching services for families that need to learn to care for their elderly relatives.

Will these specialized geriatric programs and services become realities or are they merely daydreams? The answer lies partially with the senior citizens of today. These people are beginning to effect a change in attitudes and approaches to the aged and aging. Perhaps the desired changes will not take place immediately, but the efforts of these people may have a profound effect on what tomorrow will bring for their children and grandchildren.

Citizens over sixty form an active and a powerful political group. They can constitute a major voting bloc—a real voting power. They are not afraid to make their wishes known, either in the ballot box or in demonstrations at state and federal legislative sessions. Truly, these people are not sitting passively in a rocking chair. Rather they are rocking the boat in their demands for reform, recognition, and fair treatment. This political power is known as "senior power." The most militant wing of this group, the Gray Panthers, is pledged to sit-downs, picketing, sit-ins, and other forms of demonstration until the needs of the elderly have been met.

When senior power is combined with nursing power, perhaps we can begin to attain the goal of the better life and better nursing care for our elderly citizens. This is a worthwhile investment, because eventually we will be the recipients of the benefits.

STUDY QUESTIONS AND PROBLEMS

1. Many nurses move from city to city and from job to job and are unable to transfer earned pension credits from institution to institution. Investigate other methods of preparing for economic security during retirement.
2. What leisure activities are you now engaged in that could be utilized constructively during your retirement years?
3. Imagine yourself as a retired person. What services would you find most necessary? Are such services currently available in your community? If not, what role could you play in developing them?

BIBLIOGRAPHY

de Beauvoir, Simone. *The Coming of Age.* New York: G. P. Putnam's Sons, 1972.

Laas, William. *Helpful Hints on Managing Your Money for Retirement.* New York: Popular Library, 1970.

————. *1971 White House Conference on Aging.* A Report to the Delegates from the Conference Sections and Special Concerns Sessions. Washington, D.C.: U. S. Government Printing Office, 1971.

Toffler, Alvin. *Future Shock.* New York: Bantam Books, 1970.

Townsend, Claire, project director. *Old Age: The Last Segregation.* New York: Grossman, 1971.

Service Agencies

Administration on Aging
Social Security Administration
Department of Health, Education, and Welfare
Washington, D.C. 20025

American Association of Retired Persons
National Headquarters
1225 Connecticut Avenue, N.W.
Washington, D.C. 20036

American Nursing Home Association
Suite 607
1025 Connecticut Avenue
Washington, D.C. 20036

American Psychiatric Association
1700 18th Street, N.W.
Washington, D.C. 20009

Institute of Lifetime Learning
American Association of Retired Persons
DuPont Circle Building
Washington, D.C. 20036

Institute of Lifetime Learning
American Association of Retired Persons
215 Long Beach Boulevard
Long Beach, California 90802

International Society of Laryngectomees
219 E. 42nd Street
New York, New York 10017

Mature Temps
American Association of Retired Persons
521 Fifth Avenue
New York, New York 10017

Peace Corps
Washington, D.C. 20025

United Ostomy Association
1111 Wilshire Boulevard
Los Angeles, California 90017

VISTA
Washington, D.C. 20025

Index

Page numbers in *italics* indicate illustrations.

Nervous system diseases, restorative nursing for, 131–154. See also names of specific diseases.
Nocturnal frequency, 41
Nutrition, during rehabilitation, 73
for diabetes mellitus, 181
for disoriented patient, 146

Occupational therapy, as part of rehabilitation, 82
Older adults. See specific entries.
Older Americans Act, 30
Osteoarthritis, 114

Paraffin wax baths, in treatment of arthritis, 110
Parkinson's disease, 131–138
course of, 138
diagnosis of, 132
drugs used in treatment of, 133
incidence, 131
nursing considerations for, 134
onset, 131
symptoms, 131
treatment of, 133
Patients, bedridden. See *Bedridden patients.*
elderly, diversional activities for, 93
individual care for, 57
Peace Corps, employment of retired persons in, 14
Pension, income from, 15
Personal hygiene, during rehabilitation, 88
Personality changes, in aging, 3
Physical therapy, as part of rehabilitation, 82
Pronation, exercises for, 67
Prone positioning, for hemiplegic patient, *164*
Prosthesis, hip, procedure of, 121
preparation for weight bearing, *126*
Protein, loss of, during inactivity, 73
Public housing, for senior citizens, 26
Pull-up device, *84*
Pulmonary disease, chronic obstructive, 171. See entries under *Emphysema.*

Quad cane, use of, *170*

Range of motion, maintaining, 65
Range-of-motion exercises, 66, 67, *68, 69*
for hemiplegic patient, 165
Reaction time, slowing of, with age, 46
Rehabilitation. See also under names of specific disorders.
acquiring independence during, 78
adequate nutrition during, 73

Rehabilitation, *cont.*
after amputation, 123
after hip fracture, 121, 122
ambulation during, 94
eating activities during, 92
elimination problems during, 76
encouragement during, 79
exercises for, 67
loss of protein during, 73
modification of home environment, 102
Parkinson's disease, 134
personal hygiene during, 88
physical therapy in, 82
preparation for hospital discharge, 100
prevention of decubitus ulcers during, 71
prevention of deformity during, 70
prevention of respiratory complications during, 71
self-care activities, 78
weight-reduction during, 74
Rehabilitation nursing, 62–80. See also under specific disorders.
Rehabilitation program, active, 63
candidates for, 64
roles of nursing personnel, 64
Remarriage, 23
Remotivation technique, 151
Respiratory changes, in aging, 36
Respiratory-circulatory diseases, restorative nursing for, 155–178. See also names of specific diseases.
Respiratory complications, prevention of, during rehabilitation, 71
Restorative nursing, 62–80. See also under specific areas and disorders.
Retirement, 13–21
adjustment to, 13
changing residence during, 17
club activities during, 14
education during, 15
for single adult, 24
health care costs during, 19
in future, 214–216
income during, 15
adjustment to, 17
part-time employment during, 13
planning for, 215
readjustment of couple to each other during, 19
remarriage during, 23
effect on Social Security payments, 24
shopping considerations during, 18
volunteer work during, 14
Rheumatoid arthritis, 107
characteristics of, 107
treatment for, 108